The Grand Unified Theory of Weight Loss

Ben Wilson

Ben Wilson Publishing

Amazon Kindle Direct Publishing

Copyright © 2020 Ben Wilson

Cover Design by Chris Bicourt

Paperback

ISBN: 9781838325701

CONTENTS

Introduction ix

Section 1: Before the Transformation – What They Forgot To
Teach You or Simply Lied to You About.................................**1**

    Start Believing in the Impossible...................................3

    Acknowledge Your Trajectory...11

    Divide by Three...15

    Stop Believing These Lies...17

    Solve the Body Positivity Dilemma...............................23

    Recognise Your Feelings Around Change...................29

    Clarify What You Can Actually Improve.....................33

    Remember You Are Not Alone.......................................41

    Drop Your Story..47

    Accept What Really Creates Change...........................49

    Understand How Feelings & Behaviours Change......51

Section 2: The Mechanics of Physical Change **63**

How Do You Lose Fat...65

The Practical View of How to Lose Fat..........................68

How Do You Gain Muscle..111

How Do You Change Posture.......................................135

How Do You Develop Optimal Health.......................141

How Do You Develop Your Fitness.............................149

How To Improve Your Emotional Well-being..........157

Managing Focus & Accepting Limitations.................163

Section 3: The Grand Unified Theory of Body
Transformations...**169**

Why A Grand Unified Theory......................................171

The Results Process..173

Grand Unified Theory of Body Transformations......179

The Transformation Cycle Overview...........................181

The Grand Unified Theory in Action..........................185

The Start of The Transformation Cycle......................191

Taking Action & Avoiding Procrastination.................203

The Core of the Transformation Cycle.......................217

The Change Techniques Explained.............................293

Section 4: Your Grand Unified Transformation Plan..............**331**

The Art of the Body Transformation..........................333

Approaches to Change..334

Transformation Plans..341

Before You Start Any Plan...343

The Master Plan – 26 Week Transformation...........347

The Express Master Plan – 12 Weeks........................389

The Master Plan +Plus – 26 Weeks...........................391

The Targeted Techniques Plan...................................397

Your Personalised Plan...401

Troubleshooting Q&A..403

References & Resources...416

Ben Wilson – Author Biography.................................441

Dedication

This book is dedicated to my Mother Vanessa Wilson who passed away in 2018.

Acknowledgements

I would like to thank the many people who have influenced me over the last decade as I brought this concept together. This includes friends, family, training partners, mentors, coaches as well as researchers across the many different disciplines that contributed to this.

A special thanks to my clients who were willing guinea pigs with many of the concepts and techniques presented here.

A big shout out to my friends Chris Bicourt, James Cheeseman, Gemma Mercurio and Selma Prado who supported me during the process. Finally, I would like to thank my family; Clive, Jo and Saul.

Introduction

This book is about helping you get out of the weight loss trap and changing your body both inside and out. It is the most comprehensive approach to weight loss that you will see and you will learn exactly what you need to do achieve your goals.

It will help you break your old patterns and achieve something that for many seems impossible. However, the answer does not lie in some magic diet plan, exercise routine or set of affirmations. It lies within a broader, more comprehensive model. This book will show you how to use this approach. It works for anyone, regardless of your circumstances or history. Therefore it will work for you!

How Did We Get Here?

I am not sure if there is a less successful industry in the world than the 'weight loss business'. The majority of the population want to improve their body shape and most will try to lose weight at some point. However, only a tiny percentage make any meaningful progress and even less actually maintain these results long term.

I am sure you have no doubt experienced this process; you try to lose weight and fail. Eventually you find the energy to try again yet achieve the same disappointing results. Perhaps you make progress on one attempt but then slowly creep back to where you started. You feel bad about it, blame yourself for failing and decide to give up trying. However, before you know it, you are back giving it one more attempt..... The cycle continues!

Adding insult to injury, you are probably completely confused about what to do. Every single bit of advice has someone saying the exact opposite. Some of the advice has worked for you, most of it has not. Often the approach that has worked for you before has also failed you at other times.

The only logical solution you come to is that losing weight is not realistic and it is just impossible… "I cannot do it!" the voice screams in your head. The weight loss industry would not like to admit it but that is the most logical conclusion you could take from all of your experiences.

However, there is one nagging bit of evidence that stops you truly accepting this doomed fate. That is, you know someone who has changed their body and maintained the results. You have also read, watched or heard many stories of people just like you or in a significantly worse situation achieve the most ridiculous, jaw dropping body transformations and they also sustained it afterwards.

A Better Way Forward?

You do not have to be trapped in a cycle of failure, you can change. While only a small percentage succeed, a small percentage of a huge number of people trying means hundreds of thousands of people have been very successful. So what is it that separates the successful from the majority who fail? The Grand Unified Theory of Weight Loss will answer this question.

It will provide you with a long term solution so that you can change your body now yet in a way you can maintain the results going forwards. You will learn and understand what you need to do to create change and also what you can stop doing from your previous ineffective approaches.

You will see just how much potential you have, how you are not doomed to a life of deterioration and regression but growth and success. You will learn how to extract this potential from within.

The majority of things you will read in the book will be completely new to you because you never have learnt about changing your body through the perspective of developing you and your behaviours.

The weight loss industry focuses exclusively on the plan but long term results are first about YOU and then the plan that you follow. The Grand Unified Theory of Weight Loss works on both aspects.

By the end of the process you will find it laughable how you used to blame yourself for not being able to follow your plan of action. Instead you will feel proud of the results you achieve and your ability to maintain them. You can also do all of this while living a life where you are not controlled by your weight, eating habits or thoughts around food or your body.

A Holistic Transformation – My definition

The results you want are much more than just losing weight. You are more than how much body fat you have or how much muscle you are carrying around. Any change in external shape needs to come alongside having robust health, optimal fitness and excellent mental wellbeing.

While much of these additional changes will improve as a welcome side benefit of changing your body shape it is important to check you are achieving a holistic transformation. In our obsession to change the outside we can often forget what is inside.

Physical and mental wellbeing involves feeling good about your body and yourself. It is about being free from obsessions, worry or guilt around how you look, how you eat or your exercise routine.

For this reason the true name of the method you are about to learn is actually the 'Grand Unified Theory of Body Transformations'. This includes all things weight loss of course, but also everything else such as gaining muscle, changing posture, developing fitness, increasing health and changing your mental and emotional perspectives. These elements comprise a true holistic transformation.

How to Use This Book

The book has four sections. The first section is very important because you probably have gaps in your fundamental knowledge around creating change. If this is not corrected you may never be able to progress.

In the second section you will learn everything you need to know about the mechanics of change at a physical level. How to lose fat, gain muscle or change your posture. It also includes how to achieve the other holistic goal elements.

The third section will teach you about the Grand Unified Theory of Body Transformations and how to use it to achieve your goals. It will become clear why you have struggled previously and what you need to develop going forwards. It shows you how to implement the actions outlined in section two into the real world by changing your behaviours, forming habits and handling the stresses of everyday living.

The final section has plans for you to follow. There are different approaches to use and you will learn which one would be best for you. It has all the details you will need to follow the plan and get great results.

****

Kate, 24 – Even though she was young she had been dieting for over a decade. She had lost and gained maybe 30kg in that time. She was anorexic for a period while in school and suffered with bulimia at other times. When she came to me she was still suffering from binge eating and had an awful relationship with food. She hated her body and refused to ever be in a photo. She was single and her relationships were by her own admission a disaster, mainly because of her own insecurities. She had done every diet invented and exercised all the time to burn off what she was eating.

The conventional approach would see Kate repeat the weight loss / weight gain cycle perhaps for the rest of her life. She would try a diet plan or exercise scheme and make progress. Then she would regress, feel guilty and repeat over and over.

What worked for Kate was realising that she was stuck in this endless cycle and using her frustration at the situation to finally break free. I suggested to her we should first look into her body image before trying to change her actual body. This may seem counter intuitive but when she eased up a little on her self-hatred she was able to take a more relaxed approach to change. This meant she was then able to address her binge eating. Within a fairly short period of time she felt really good about herself even though her body was the same as before.

At this point it was surprisingly easy to learn how to lose body fat slowly and gently. Albeit there were a few setbacks along the way she was much more forgiving when these happened. In the end she managed to achieve her goals both externally and internally. She got to her goal weight and actually liked the person she had become.

****

Section 1

Before The Transformation – What They Forgot To Teach You or Simply Lied to You About

To be successful you need to have a solid understanding on a variety of fundamentals. The health and fitness arena is difficult because you would have learnt many things that are incorrect which are now blocking your progress. Therefore, if you want to proceed you will need to unlearn these.

Health & Fitness is also tricky in that there are other areas and facets you simply do not know exist. This means, you will not go out and learn about it because you do not know it is even there. This again limits your progress going forwards.

This section therefore fills any gaps in your knowledge, breaks down blocks to progress and ensures You and I are both on the same wavelength going forwards.

Start Believing in the 'Impossible'

We shall start your transformation with a look at the very base foundation of change, which is your belief in the possibility that you can succeed.

This day and age most people do not believe they can actually change their body and even if they could they would not be able to maintain the results. It is understandable with the amount of times you have probably tried and failed previously that you may have a large set of limiting beliefs around your ability to be successful.

However, you are wrong, change is possible, you can change on the outside and you can change on the inside. You can change how you think, how you act and how you feel about all aspects related to your health & fitness. You can also easily maintain your results for the rest of your life.

There are many reasons why you may think change is impossible. This could relate to the physical body itself, whether you could ever lose your bad habits or perhaps you question if you have the motivation to put in the necessary effort. Let me show you why none of these are true.

Physical Impossibility

You may feel that you are stuck with your weight due to your metabolism, age, genetics, hormones or other health related issues. This is understandable however, have you considered any of the following scenarios and how it would affect you:

- **Famine** – If a famine was to strike the country today and food shortages began it would mean you could no longer freely graze on food. You would eat only what you could get your hands on. With inadequate amounts of food around what would happen to you and everyone in the population? There are only two options, you would either lose weight or you would become ill from malnutrition and die. We know this is true because when famines occur around the world people do not gain weight, they lose it. Whenever the government has enforced food rations (during wartimes) the population loses body fat at predictable speeds.

- **'Prison' Shed Experiments** – While we rarely have famine in the western world, what would happen if I recreated those conditions in your life. Imagine if I locked you in a shed with a bed and a treadmill. What would happen if I forced you to walk a certain distance to be fed and then gave you only limited amounts of food as a reward? You would hate me for it but you would lose fat none the less. This has been shown in medical ward dieting studies when people are not allowed to leave the room so all food is controlled. A five star version of this can be seen with high end detox retreats. You pay a lot of money to be put in very nice hotel & spa but also to be limited to 600 calories a day. These retreats produce predictable fat loss and stay in business despite the cost.

- **What Goes Up Must Come Down** – Do you accept you can gain weight? Almost everyone I have ever asked acknowledges that they will gain fat fairly easily if they let their behaviours go a little. If that is the case then this shows the fat accumulation process is working normally. If it is working in regards to gaining fat then it must be working normally for losing fat as well. It cannot only go in one direction. If you can gain it, you can lose it. This means weight loss is possible if you create the right conditions.

- **Brain Swap** – What would happen if someone of great fitness who is good at losing weight brain swapped into your body? What if not just swapping brains but you also swapped lifestyles? Though the new person in your body would initially need to adjust to the new environment it is unlikely that someone who has been exercising every day for years with balanced nutrition would all of a sudden stop moving and start eating junk food. On the flipside, if you were brain swapped into a professional athletes or fitness model's body would you have the knowledge, skills or motivation to keep their results and standards?

- **You Already Have Lost Weight** – How many times have you lost weight already? Almost everyone has lost weight at some point in their life even if just for a couple of weeks before returning back to your old habits. If you have lost weight before it shows that physically at least, it is possible again.

*****

The above elements show that it is not a physical issue per se, or a block in your physiology that is the reason you cannot lose body fat. If you were forced into the right conditions for fat loss you would lose weight. However, in the real world you are free to act however you would like. This means your results are determined by your ability to stick to the behaviours that create fat loss.

Though everyone can lose body fat it seems fairly clear that some people have it a little harder than others. This is due to various physiological functions from hunger to metabolism. This is different to it being impossible to get results. It is just harder for some people, though whoever you are, getting into shape is never easy. The key is how you train the brain to be able do the tasks needed for results regardless of your circumstances.

Behavioural Impossibility

You may understand that it is not a physical issue per se stopping you from losing weight. However, as you are unable to change your behaviours around health & fitness in any sort of practical, meaningful way it is still effectively impossible. This viewpoint is understandable but are you really stuck with your bad behaviours? When looking at behaviour change and the possibilities of it, here are some things to consider:

- **You Know You Can Develop Bad Behaviours** – It pretty much goes without saying that you are currently able to develop bad behaviours. In fact, if you do nothing we could probably guess in a few years you will have naturally picked up some new bad habits. If you are able to develop bad behaviours then this shows the behaviour / habit creation system is still working as it should within your brain. This means it can be used to create good habits in the same way it is already creating bad ones.

- **You Already Have Developed Some Good Behaviours** – You have probably forgotten or discounted many of your current good behaviours because you are all too caught up focusing on the bad stuff you want to get rid of. If you think back in your life what good behaviours have you created previously? Maybe you used to smoke but you stopped, perhaps you used to drink a lot more than you do currently, did you take up exercise or start eating vegetables? Almost everyone can find examples of good behaviours they have created at some point in their life. If you have done it before, it means you can do it now. The behaviour creation pathway worked then and it will work now.

- **Your Life Story is littered with Behaviour Change** – If you look back on your life it is basically one long story of behaviour change. It shows you following certain behaviours for a while, struggling with others and forming new habits throughout your life. There is no question about whether you can change your behaviour because your life is constantly changing. The real issue is to understand how to manage change to be more in favour of the areas you are looking to improve. Body transformations are just a series of small behaviours that need modifying.

An Impossible Effort

If you accept that physically it is possible to achieve you goals and that behaviour change could happen however unlikely it may seem, then you are a long way towards having enough belief to move forwards. Do not worry if you do not know how to do this yet, we are just getting started.

The next area most people struggle with is a belief that the process is just too much effort, even though it could happen in theory you are not the kind of person who has the motivation to do so. You probably think you could not put in the needed effort for long enough to get results. It is helpful to consider the following:

- **The Effort of Not Changing** – Often you are so focused on finding the energy to change you lose track of how much effort you are unnecessarily wasting within your current lifestyle. When you are not at your goal it usually means you are suffering lower energy or feel worse than you should and waste a lot of time worrying about your situation. When overweight or out of shape it takes an extra effort just to do the normal things in life.

The habits of eating badly, drinking too much or not exercising drain the life, energy and confidence from you. While it does take some effort to create change it is a deception to think where you are currently is a bed of roses. If you change nothing going forwards then your current life will take more and more effort just to maintain it.

- **Previous Efforts in Life** – You have already put in more than enough effort to achieve your health & fitness goals at various points of your life. This could have been specifically with your body in previous transformations or from the struggle of following a really bad plan of action day in, day out. A bad plan will drain your effort yet gives you none of the rewards. It is very common to see this happen.

Even if you have had zero success with your body you would have put in enough effort within other areas of your life. This could be when you were studying, within your career, dealing with your children, getting through periods of high stress or simply living with difficult life circumstances. That same ability still lies within you even if you have lost touch with the resource in recent times. If that energy is directed into your goal with the right approach you will be pleasantly surprised about your potential and abilities to get stuff done.

- **Your Current Efforts Now in the Wrong Places** – Very often you are putting in enough effort at this current moment. In this case it is simply about directing your energy into more productive outcomes. Perhaps you are focusing on extra reps rather than creating new behaviours, maybe you are trying to eat tuna and broccoli all day over finding a nutrition scheme that tastes great and gets results. It is a real waste to see people not getting results because their effort is being badly misdirected but it commonly happens.

Impossible To Sustain

If you understand that it is not just possible but more than realistic to change your behaviours you may start worrying whether the results are at all sustainable, why go through all this to just put it back on? In this case it may be helpful to consider the following:

- **Current Maintenance** – Most people have been at their current weight or body shape for a long time already, perhaps for a few months or often many years. In this case you have shown how easy it is to maintain your current physique. It takes no more effort to maintain a better level of body shape. All that is missing is the focused period to change from where you are today to where you want to be. Once there it can be maintained just like you are already doing, this includes all the bad behaviours you are doing today. These can be done to maintain your goal body in the future.

- **Previous Maintenance** – It could be that you lost weight before but put that back on as the years have passed by. It can be a little unfair to say that this is an issue of unsustainability. Very often when you look into your history, you changed your body then kept it off for a fairly long period of time, perhaps many months or even years. Then at some point you started to gain weight. It is important to remember how you maintained that shape fairly easily for such a long time before regaining the weight.

- **Physiological Demands of Maintenance** – If you have gone through a body transformation then you have more than enough of everything to maintain your results. To maintain your body is much easier than changing it, you can eat more food, move less, train less and still stay where you are. It is easier to maintain than progress in all areas when looking at it from a physiological demand point of view.

Why You Need to Start Believing

Truth be told, you do not need to actually believe in success to get results, you just need to do the necessary actions. However, in reality, you will do hardly any of these actions if you do not have some element of hope in the potential of getting results.

It is more than possible to achieve your goals. There are no actual physical blocks to success and you can easily change your behaviours if you use the right approach. This can all be done with a sensible level of effort and in a way that you could maintain your results for the rest of your life.

I don't expect you to believe everything I have just said despite it being true. I know you have a collection of negative past experiences around trying to change your body. All you need to understand is that getting results is within the realms of possibility. You do not need to truly believe it will happen, but understand that it could happen. For example, you know it is possible you could win the lottery and it is this hope that gets you buying your ticket.

The odds of getting in shape are vastly better than winning any lottery, especially as success is completely under your own control and not left to luck. So you only need to have a little hope and belief in the possibility of what could happen to move forwards.

***** Questions to Consider *****

-What are your current beliefs around the probability of you losing weight?

-If you knew that it was possible to get results how would you act differently going forwards?

Acknowledge Your Trajectory

It is helpful to understand the path that you have been on up until this point and what that means for the future.

Where Are You Today and Why?

Where you are today in terms of health and fitness, both internally and externally is the total summation of your previous experiences.

At a surface level it is the result of what you have been eating and how much you have been moving over the past months to years. At another level, it is the representation of how you react to hunger and how you feel emotionally about food and exercise. On an even deeper level it is the interaction of memories and emotions that have been built upon by thousands of repeated behaviours, actions and experiences.

The surface level seems to be where the fitness industry is stuck, "Just eat less and move more…. It is so simple to do… LOOK AT ME!..." goes the average fitness expert. To analyse results at this level is to do a disservice to you, to them and everyone involved in the change process. The Grand Unified Theory of Body Transformations goes way beyond this basic and somewhat insulting standard of interpretation.

However, the mantra runs deep within most people. Every week I have a client standing before me feeling guilty, upset or in tears because they feel they have 'failed'. Perhaps they had some chocolate, a few glasses of wine or didn't exercise as planned. The problem is not the behaviours, it is the expectations they hold. You cannot discount your past and assume it has no influence upon you going forwards.

What has gone before influences how you will act now and also how fast it will be to create change. For example, take exercise adherence, the average fitness expert has enjoyed exercise since they were a child and there is a good chance they have had 5000+ positive exercise experiences by the time they reach adulthood. If you have never liked exercising then you may have had just a few positive experiences with fitness if any. It is therefore not a fair fight to wonder why you are so "bad" with exercise consistency and your fitness guru is so "great". Going forwards you need an approach that accounts for your personal background.

Where Will You Be Tomorrow and Why?

Your behaviours over recent months to years have created your physical results today and these behaviours were formed from your experiences, feelings and actions in the past. So what of the future?

As you go forwards, certain things are guaranteed to happen; you will get older, society will influence you in many ways both positive and negative, you will go through change (new jobs, relationships etc.) and you will go through stress (arguments, bereavement and so forth). These changes will test your current behaviour patterns further.

Due to our modern lifestyles it is more likely you will become lazier over time rather than more active. It is also more likely you will eat larger food portions than smaller ones if left to your own devices. This means if you do nothing, your health & fitness will probably decline going forwards.

How Do You Create a Different Tomorrow?

It is more than possible to change your projected path going forwards. This book is about showing you how to do that. The key is to not leave it to chance. While it is possible that something will inspire change and suddenly you transform in a positive direction, it is not commonplace or expected. As mentioned, the opposite is likely, your fitness gets worse, your weight increases and eating habits deteriorate. The way to prevent this is by making a conscious decision to change and improve your health & fitness.

***** Questions to Consider *****

-What have been your experiences (good/bad) with the following?

-Exercise
-Healthy Eating
-Junk Foods
-Trying to change your body

-Based on your past experiences and life up until now what is the likely outcome of your body going forwards?

Divide By Three

It is essential to understand the difference between YOUR BEHAVIOURS, YOUR BODY and the YOU who is reading this book. This is because your body and your behaviours act automatically and have many actions going on that are not under your control. It is like they have a mind of their own.

When you confuse yourself for your body or behaviours it sets you up for disappointment and frustration. You will blame yourself for mistakes and be angry about your struggles to get results. This is unnecessary because it assumes you are calmly in control of all of your actions, in reality the body or your behaviours will often lead you. At other times you lead them.

Examples of this interplay include when you binge eat because of low blood sugar (body), if you eat badly only when around friends (behaviour) or when you cut out junk food and resist cravings at the start of a new regime (You).

A good analogy of this process is to think about riding a horse. The horse represents your body and behaviours while you are the jockey. However good you are at riding you are never totally in charge of the process, the horse still has a mind of its own. For many people when they try to change shape it is like they are on a very unruly horse for the first time ever. It can take time to learn how to ride and direct the animal but with practice anyone can become skilled at it.

***** Questions to consider *****

-Can you think of times where your body seemed to take control over your actions?

-Can you think of times where your automatic behaviours / habits seemed to take over your actions?

Stop Believing These Lies!

There are a few major myths that almost everyone, including you, probably believes. This is because you have been lied to about it year upon year. This misinformation results in you putting your focus into the wrong areas and in a way that is not at all tailored to you. As a result you fail over and over and end up thinking it is impossible to achieve your goals.

NOT TRUE - Transformations Are About Knowledge

Getting in shape or changing your body is <u>not</u> about knowledge. This is where the weight loss and health & fitness industry are stuck. They keep selling you plans with knowledge on it under the misassumption that it is a lack of knowledge that prevents you from being successful. Year after year of this you now are so confused you do not know what to believe. This conveniently allows another person to sell you a solution with yet more knowledge.

Forget knowledge! This whole section of the book is mostly about trying to get you to forget a lot of what you know. You know too much! This information overload drowns out the actual facts you need and distracts you from focusing on what really gets results. Success in body transformations come from your skills and not knowledge.

A skill is an applied, practiced and rehearsed behaviour that you do in the real world. Almost everything around being successful in creating a new body is based on your skill levels and <u>not</u> what information you store in your brain.

For example, you know you should go and exercise this evening (knowledge) but it takes something else to go out and actually do it (the skill to get yourself to exercise). You know you should stop eating that packet of biscuits (knowledge) but it takes a clever approach to actually put them away (skills around eating). It is easy to say go for a walk and meditate when stressed (knowledge) but takes a different way of thinking to actually do it when emotions are running high (skills under a certain emotional state).

The characterisation of a body transformation as being about knowledge instead of skills is one of the most fundamental errors of the whole weight loss industry.

If you did think of developing skills over knowledge you would immediately take a very different approach to your transformations. Everyone understands learning a skill, no one would pick up a guitar and expect to be able to play like a rock star within an hour.

I could tell you how to drive a car in about 3 minutes but it takes many hours of practice to do it at a basic level and many more hours to be able to do it on the roads or under the pressure of a driving test. Using a skill based approach you will have more patience and know it takes repetitions to be successful.

NOT TRUE - Transformations Are About Effort

All anyone mentions when it comes to getting in shape is how they wish they had more motivation, more willpower or could try a little bit harder. On the surface it appears that this is what is separating you from achieving results but it is a lie.

Motivation does not vary as much as you would think between those who are successful with their goals and those who are not. What separates people are their automatic behaviours (how they respond without thinking) and their skill levels (how many times they have practiced a specific behaviour). These elements are developed from consistency over time rather than effort or motivation.

It is duration and persistence that separates those who are successful from those who struggle. If the weight loss industry talked about how to sustain behaviours instead of motivating you to go harder you would get much better results.

Do you need motivation to develop persistence? Yes and no, the traditional approach of motivation as promoted in the weight loss industry is not needed. This is when you get motivated and put all that energy into actions to get results today. You do a hard exercise session, cut out all bad foods, try to lose weight quickly etc. This does not work for most people.

A more effective approach is to use any surge in motivation to direct it into actions that would significantly enhance your chances of longer term changes within your behaviours.

Instead of doing some really hard exercise sessions you could commit to trying five new types of exercise. This increases your chances of finding an activity you may enjoy rather than hoping you will somehow fall in love with an exercise type you have already been inconsistent with.

A better avenue than cutting out all bad foods would be learning to become a better chef. A seven day challenge to cooking a new healthy recipe every day would be more successful than going hard on a salad only diet.

A more effective approach than trying to lose as much weight as possible in 14 days would be to ask yourself how many weeks do you truly need to get to your goal, then plan this while accounting for off periods and breaks within it. This could be the difference between trying every year to lose weight and actually succeeding.

It is no surprise that few people do this. You have been sold a plan on effort and the thought of doing that for anything more than a few days let alone a few weeks is a hard sell. However this is yet another misconception. When you do things focused on duration it is much easier than you thought. Almost all of the worst bits of getting in shape stem from the emphasis on effort and going hard on your plan.

It could be that you are thinking this is all fair enough but I just want to change my body quickly then get back to my normal life. This is how most people think, give me the results ASAP. The problem is that it doesn't work long term.

You do need some motivation, it is one of the key areas within the Grand Unified Theory of Body Transformations. However, the motivation is needed so you commit for a longer duration with a focus on developing you. It is not so that you try harder hoping for fast results while trying to be the exact same person as before.

NOT TRUE - Transformations Are All The Same

The difficulty of any transformation varies greatly between people as does the steps and actions you need to take. Yet the underlying lie is that body transformations are effectively the same for everyone.

This is seen across the weight loss industry where everyone flocks to the guy or girl in great shape because they must know how to do it. However, this thought process negates your whole personal history and crushes any individual considerations around your own body.

There are so many factors that can vary between you and someone else. One of the most obvious is simply the change needed based on your current natural habits. To achieve your goal you will need to do certain behaviours, if you already do those behaviours then you do not need to think about it at all. If you are not doing them then you will need to develop them.

You see this example all the time when people try to copy the exercise plans of those in great shape, if you exercise once a week if lucky and they train every day all year round then you are not the same. You need a plan to improve your exercise consistency. If you follow a plan based on liking exercise already you will probably fail.

This is why so many people who are trying to get in shape are following some form of a plan that professional body builders use. The methods they employ have flooded the advice and recommendations to get in shape because they have the most muscle and least body fat. However, this has little to no application to 95% of people out there who have more normal goals and a typical background around food and exercise.

If you drink yet I do not, your transformation plan will need to consider this factor. If you want to drop a dress size yet I want to gain 10kg of muscle to be on the front of a fitness magazine, the difficulty, dedication and duration needed for us is not the same.

Individuality stems not just from changing your current habits to the necessary ones for success but also encompasses your prior history. How you used to act still has an influence upon the changes you make today.

If you used to be an athlete and do sport in your twenties you will be able to get back into a fitness routine quicker than if you have never done exercise in your life. In both scenarios you can achieve results but you will need a slightly different approach to get there. The same applies to food, drink and how you socialise. Doing something for a second time is different to doing something for the first time. Neither is better or worse but rather you must understand all body transformations are not the same.

This is also true in the difficulty of a transformation. The more natural behaviours you need to develop the longer it will take. The bigger your goals, the longer and more focus it will take. It is simply more difficulty for some people to get results over others due to biochemistry and a host of other factors.

This means you cannot just follow advice from some guy who happens to be in shape. You need a plan that covers what is blocking you from succeeding with the patience and the specificity to develop this plan over time.

***** Questions to Consider *****

-To what extent have you believed the three lies outlined?

-How have they affected your behaviours to get in shape?

Solve the Body Positivity Dilemma

Before we delve into the many aspects around body shape and change there is an important conversation to be had around body positivity. An imbalance on this topic will make it hard to impossible to achieve your goals.

Body Positivity

The premise behind this philosophy is that everyone deserves to have a positive body image regardless of what shape they are in, all bodies are acceptable and a pathway to good self-esteem. The movement looks to break free from the narrow cultural classifications of 'Good' vs 'Bad' body shapes and that no particular body type should be used to define the ideal. There are some great elements to this philosophy that you must encompass for success.

However, the extreme end of this viewpoint is that you do not need to change anything. It is often assumed in the theory that when you become free from judgement you will choose to do the best things for you, your health and your body. However, this frequently is not the case.

Traditional Goals Setting

The traditional approach to your body has been to set a goal and go for it. The silent implication behind this is where you are today is 'bad'. It assumes you should aim for your ideal weight and that you will feel better when you get there. This approach is still the most prevailing amongst society. While it has benefits it can also bring problems and impede progress.

Body Positivity vs Goal Setting

These two approaches to changing your body have created a mini war between the followers of each side. There have been many arguments, debates and TV chat shows jumping on the topic. It created hostility between people who believe you should change your body and strive to be an ideal weight and those who feel you should love yourself as you are and do not need to change anything.

In reality, the controversy of body positivity shined a light on a bigger question, how should you feel about area any area of your life you could change? Should you try to improve it or focus on feeling content? There are no right or wrong answers to this question.

I do not believe there is any reason to make this an either / or issue. There is no reason to hate yourself, you can love yourself as you are yet there is also nothing wrong with being excited about wanting to achieve something in the area of your body shape.

This shows itself all across our lives, for example, you do not have to hate your job to want to progress your career and change roles within it. Likewise, you do not have to hate where you live to want to go on holiday somewhere nice. It is perfectly fine to appreciate and like where you are yet still have a deep motivation and excitement towards a goal.

A Personal Choice

I believe it is a personal decision if you want to change your body. You get to decide how to live your life. I have never told someone they need to lose weight. It is not my place to do so.

The key to making wise choices is being aware of the consequences of how any decision may affect your body and your life in general. For example, if someone chooses to smoke then that is fine, however it is important they know the likely consequences of doing this and have help available if they decide to quit. The same applies around your body.

Body Positivity vs The Best for You

If you make 'doing the best for you as a person', as the basis for making decisions the traditional views of goal setting align with the body positivity movement.   What is best for you is a balance between fulfilling your short-term desires and wishes vs any longer term consequences. For example, it is fun to do a bit of clothes shopping but spending all of your money today will result in stress and unhappiness in the longer term. Staying in bed feels good but being sacked for not going to work would bring negative consequences.

As well as the short term pleasure you would want to also factor in the longer term benefits to any decision. Eliminating junk food out of the diet may bring temporary discomfort but longer term means you feel better, happier and more energised every single day. Likewise, to start an exercise plan may be hard but you will feel happier overall as an exerciser.

When you consider the deeper feelings alongside the short term it allows for more sensible decisions to be made. It isn't about whether to choose short vs long term, but rather how you balance them both.

Body Positivity Vs Your Subconscious

It is also important to clarify the consistency between what you say and what you believe subconsciously. There is a difference in what you would like to believe and what you actually do believe at an emotional / behavioural level.

The simplest way to look into this is through examining your emotions. For example, you could say, "Anyone should be able to eat whatever they want and enjoy food" yet when you eat chocolate you feel guilty about it. In this case your subconscious has a different rule set to what you would like to consciously believe.

The same can happen with your body image. You say that you like yourself exactly how you are yet emotionally you are not confident enough to do certain things because of the way you look. The longer term goal would be to align your subconscious and conscious beliefs together. You can change your subconscious through looking at your current system of evaluation, where it came from and more effective methods.

The Goal Setting vs Body Positivity Balance Scales

This whole debate can be summed up if you view the two approaches as weights on a counterbalance. The most effective way forwards is to ensure you are balanced between the two views. If you lean too far in either direction, be it towards a goals centred approach or a body positivity perspective it will bring undue consequences for you. The two sides of the scale can be summed by;

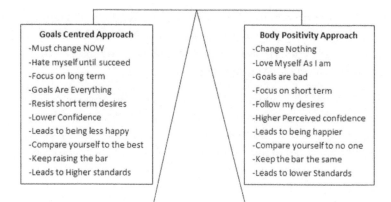

Goals Centred Approach	Body Positivity Approach
-Must change NOW	-Change Nothing
-Hate myself until succeed	-Love Myself As I am
-Focus on long term	-Goals are bad
-Goals Are Everything	-Focus on short term
-Resist short term desires	-Follow my desires
-Lower Confidence	-Higher Perceived confidence
-Leads to being less happy	-Leads to being happier
-Compare yourself to the best	-Compare yourself to no one
-Keep raising the bar	-Keep the bar the same
-Leads to Higher standards	-Leads to lower Standards

The extreme end of a full goal centred approach means you hate where you are, who you are and know you must change NOW! You focus on setting and achieving long term goals while sacrificing short term pleasures. You do not feel great about yourself and you are not happy as you know you can be so much more. As you progress you continue to look at higher and more difficult goals. You compare yourself to people who are better than you. In general this leads to a higher level of results but much less satisfaction with where you are today.

The extreme view of the body positivity approach means you love where you are, who you are and choose not to change anything. Your focus is on enjoying life as it with no goals for the long term. You just follow your desires. You feel great about yourself and do not need to improve anything. You only make progress with health & fitness if you happen to naturally want to eat sensibly and move. However, with no goals you have no reason to learn new health & fitness skills and with no one to compare yourself to you never understand what is possible with the body. This generally leads to a lower level of results even though you feel more satisfied with where you are today.

The best approach to take is where there is an even balance between body positivity and goal setting. You will be happy with where you are and who you are but also be excited to change and make improvements in your life.

Your focus is on longer term goals but you can also appreciate and honour short term desires in a way that does not ruin the longer term plan. You feel great about yourself because you do not need to change anything yet excited because you have decided to make improvements out of your own choice for your future self.

You are patient with progress and not in a rush to get results as soon as possible. You keep your goals the same as you progress and take inspiration from people who have 'better' results than you. You accept you do not need to be like them unless you decide it would be fun to focus on it. This ultimately leads to a higher level of results and you feel you more satisfied with where you are.

*****

It takes practice to achieve a balanced approach as it is easy to drift towards one set of beliefs. To live with this ethos you may need to investigate how you got to the point of your current beliefs. Through persistence and practice you will be able balance the scales and optimise progress forwards.

***** Questions to Consider *****

-Which end of the 'Body Positivity – Traditional Goal Setting' scale do you tend to align towards?

-What can you do to ensure you have a more balanced approach going forwards?

-What signs or markers would mean you have gone too far in either direction on the 'Body Positivity – Goals' scale?

Recognize Your Feelings Around Change

Some of the most overlooked people in the self-help or the transformation field are those who do not like the thought of change. If you do not like upheaval, trying new things or disrupting old comfortable patterns you are not alone and there is nothing wrong with this attitude.

However, if an area of your life is not where it needs to be you can find yourself trapped. Often with this viewpoint you will procrastinate greatly and find yourself only taking action when the problem is quite bad already or when it is too late, e.g. you start your diet a week before you go on holiday.

A more effective way for you to look at this issue is that change is already happening. Gradually your behaviours, fitness and health are edging in a direction you do not want them to go. This change is already in motion and you will inevitably end up in a place you dislike if you do nothing.

It is important you acknowledge these silent negative changes as they are happening to you right now. They are usually hard to spot as they are subtle and happen slowly.

In addition it is important you consider how change does not have to be how you typically imagine it. Do not get caught up in the overly hyped turn your life on its head approach the media and general society seems to promote. You can get great results making tiny subtle adjustments over time. You also do not need to stop all of your bad behaviours and can usually find a way to avoid having to do any particular actions that really do not appeal. Often the differences between a 'successful you' and a 'failing you' is just a few small changes.

Fear of Change and Safety

For many people they have very real fears about obtaining success. Some common fears include receiving unwanted attention off the opposite sex, being unable to maintain results or looking stupid if you put the weight back on. Other concerns could be people expecting you to do things differently, losing popularity with friends, changing as a person in a bad way or being singled out. These fears may be totally imagined or they could have some real merit to them, e.g. they have happened to you in the past.

Sometimes you have reservations about achieving your goal because the last time you were in shape you experienced an unrelated but very negative event, e.g. someone died, you got divorced. This will associate that negative experience with being in good shape which can create resistance to change. It could also be that your life is in such a stressed state that any change feels unsafe as you are in pure survival mode.

The way through these is to look at your fears, previous negative events and thoughts around the process. This may include using emotional management techniques as discussed later on. It may also involve looking at your overall stressors so you feel more secure. The vast majority of fears do not usually stand up when given some time and introspection and rarely happen when you actually achieve your goals.

'Away From' Motivators

Another personality trait that is usually not served by self-help is if you have an 'Away from' motivation style. This refers to people who are motivated by avoiding a problem rather than achieving a goal.

In her book "Words That Change Minds: The 14 Patterns for Mastering the Language of Influence", Sheele Rose Charvet, writes about how probably 50% of the population have this as a natural motivation style.

The fitness industry and self-help field is run by people with a 'towards focus'. That is someone who loves chasing goals and probably likes change. It makes sense really, as change based people are more likely to buy books, courses and products than 'change averse' personalities. So the circle feeds itself.

The reason this is important is that most books (including this one as it is my style) will overly stress achieving your goals and the benefits of success etc. This will not resonate with you as much as discussions of the consequences of failing to change or the problems that you are currently experiencing.

The way to maximise your motivational style is to immediately transform any talk around achieving goals into thoughts of your current problems that you want to get away from and/or the future problems you are looking to avoid.

***** Questions to Consider *****

-What aspects of change increase your procrastination and put you off from taking action?

-How have you noticed your body changing in any negative ways while not taking action?

- Imagine how you would feel at your next landmark birthday if things have got much worse than they are today?

-What negative consequences or fears do you have about achieving your goals? What could you do about these?

Clarify What You Can Actually Improve

It is important to know specifically what needs to improve to achieve your body shape goals and how to handle areas that cannot be directly changed. Too often this is an unnecessary source of confusion. The factors that influence your body shape and appearance are outlined below. These include;

Body Fat

The majority of conversations around body shape are referring to body fat. When discussing issues around weight, clothes not fitting or not liking how you look in the mirror you are usually talking about excess body fat.

You need body fat as it plays a vital role in how you function. The key is having the right amount of body fat for your ideal shape and look. As you store excess fat it makes you bigger all round as a person as well as changing the shape of your body.

Muscle Mass

The amount of muscle mass you have can totally transform the look of your physique. For many people this is a significant part of their body evaluation, especially for men.

Where you gain muscle will affect your appearance, it can make your shoulders wider, your arms thicker, waist appear thinner or change the shape of your buttocks or legs.

Being Toned – Body Fat Vs Muscle Mass

When you talk about wanting to be more toned or ripped you are referring to the balance between how much body fat you have vs the amount of muscle you have developed. The less fat you have the more toned you will look in general and likewise the more muscle you have, the more toned you will look. Therefore your goal is about the balance of these two factors. For the majority of people they will achieve their toning goals simply by losing body fat without any need to develop muscle.

A final factor to consider around toning is in relation to the stomach area. While the amount body fat vs muscle mass still applies a third factor of bloating from the digestive system also comes into consideration.

Posture

How you sit or stand affects how you look. Your posture is the most comfortable position the body adopts under gravity. Therefore, postural changes need to be made through changes in the strength, flexibility or the habitual pattern of the muscular system.

The appearance of your stomach that is not related to body fat or muscle would come under this area also. This would include bloating and stomach activation.

*****

Body fat, muscle and posture get the most of the attention in body transformation talk because they can be changed easily and obviously through nutrition & exercise programmes. However, there are other factors that affect how your body looks though most of these cannot be changed. These include the following;

Fat Distribution Pattern

This refers to where you store your body fat and it varies across the population. You could have two people with the same body fat percentage and height yet their bodies do not look the same. This is because body fat is stored in different places.

There have been a few attempts to categorize distribution patterns though none have been overly successful. The most basic is the Ectomorph, Endomorph and Mesomorph body shapes which most people are familiar with, though this is as much about muscle as it is fat.

Dr Abravanel[1] had a system using four endocrine types – Thyroid, Adrenal, Gonadal and Pituitary to classify fat storage. A textiles study[2] on body shape using 3D imaging identified eight body fat distribution patterns within women – Hourglass Shape, Bottom Hourglass Shape, Top Hourglass shape, Spoon, Rectangle, Diamond, Oval, Triangle, Inverted Triangle. There have also been other methods and theories yet none of these have really been able to either classify body shape accurately or be of any practical use.

The various body shapes occur because our fat can be stored in different places, the main issues to consider are:

- **Primary Fat Storage Areas** – This refers to where you predominantly store your body fat, e.g. on your stomach, your hips, below your waist or perhaps equally all over the whole body.

- **How Much Fat is Stored Around the Muscles** – Your body can store fat within or around the muscles. If this happens it will give you a more solid muscular look compared to someone who stores fat predominantly away from their muscles such as on their stomach or around their hips.

- **Total Amount of Body Fat You Have** - As you continue to gain fat it becomes deposited in more and more areas across the whole body. At a certain point this will start including areas that are usually lean. This could be your hands, feet, the scalp of your head and other areas. It is often hard to notice these parts gaining body fat because they will still appear leaner than the main storage areas. This will also include depositing fat around the organs (visceral fat) which the body tries to avoid doing initially due to the health consequences.

*****

The fat storage pattern you have is mostly fixed for life. It may change if there is a significant alteration in the hormonal environment, e.g. menopause, taking steroids, but in general your pattern stays the same.

Height & Bone Structure

Perhaps the very first thing you perceive is someone's height. While your height is fixed you can change how tall you appear through posture and clothes. Standing tall with your head held high makes you look taller as does dressing in one colour, using higher waisted trousers and avoiding horizontal patterns. There are many blogs detailing these methods.

Variations in bone structure will affect your appearance too. People of the same height may look different as their legs, arms, neck are not the same length.

For example, in the 2012 Olympics a report came out showing that Michel Phelps, the Gold medal swimmer who is 6 foot 4 (193 cm) had the same leg length as the Kenyan gold medallist runner who was 5 foot 10 (178cm). It was found that Michael Phelps' upper body is that of a 6 foot 8" (203cm) person[3] which is very helpful for swimming. This is genetically determined and cannot be changed.

Other Factors Affecting Appearance –

While we are looking at the factors that affect body shape this topic merges into discussions on appearance. When you look at this wider definition, of which body shape is one trait, there are many other contributing factors.

This would include facial appearance, eye colour, teeth, skin tone, skin quality and more. It would also include elements such as your clothes, fashion and style as well as your hair and even how you act. Two elements under this category which link into the body would be:

Cellulite – Many people are concerned about cellulite which relates to the surface structure of fat under the skin. It varies between individuals based on your genetics and affects both sexes though more common in women. Your cellulite becomes more pronounced and visible the higher your overall body fat and becomes less noticeable at lower body fat levels.

Breast Size – This is initially determined by genetics but it is also influenced by your body fat levels and hormones. Your breast size can change greatly as you gain or lose body fat.

What Can You Change?

The main elements to focus upon are your body fat and muscle mass. You can become smaller all round or change your body shape by losing fat. Alternatively, you can add muscle to become bigger or to change the appearance of specific body parts. There are also other aspects of appearance you can modify such as posture which has a big influence on how you look. You can also greatly change your "attractiveness" which has many elements to it outside of what is locked into your physical looks. This includes clothes, style and how you act.

What Cannot Change?

Not everything can change on your body and an undue focus on these is a guaranteed path to bad body image. Things that cannot be changed include your bone structure, your body fat distribution type and your absolute height.

Various fads and crazes within the fitness industry come back to unchangeable or unrealistic measures. The thigh gap and hip dip is massively influenced by your genetics through your bone structure. While body fat levels have some influence for most people this area cannot be changed.

Body fat patterns are genetically given, this means some people will be more naturally curvy or have a different body shape. While you can develop curves through muscle development your overall shape and body type cannot really be changed. Cellulite structure is also genetic though how pronounced it appears is affected by how much body fat you have. This means you have some control in how it looks but you can still have it even at low levels of body fat.

It is also important to remember you cannot have zero body fat. You will always have fat on your body and would die if you didn't. This means however lean you are you can always find something to grab or bend into some angle that shows you have a roll of fat. Body fat is a part of you, it is important to understand that having no body fat is <u>not</u> a possible outcome. While you may want to lose your excess fat there is no reason to hate your essential body fat.

Many people become fixated on certain aspects of their body or features that they wish they could change. This is ok if you direct it into positive action around an area that <u>can</u> change. However, it is a disaster if you focus on something that cannot be changed.

Accept What Cannot Be Changed

It is an important part of the transformation process to accept what you cannot change. This will liberate energy which can be used for focusing on what you can improve. All of this should come from a place of liking the person you are right now while being inspired to move forward.

To help this process you should look to ensure you have the right role models. Take your inspiration from people who have a similar body type and avoid focusing on an ideal that does not represent you. This can include spending less time with people who promote unhelpful beliefs within your life.

This would also include the imagery you receive from social media where you have access to anyone on the planet. Many of the people with the biggest followings have had extensive amounts of plastic surgery, body procedures or are using heavy doses of steroids. Despite this they will usually claim their look is natural and due to genetics. This can give unrealistic expectations for what you could achieve.

Success in a transformation is focused on changing the body to create a new you but it is also about relaxing the mind to accept a big part of the current you.

***** **Questions to Consider** *****

-What aspects of your body that can be changed would you like to improve?

-What can you do to start accepting the parts of your body that cannot be changed?

-Who would be a good role model for your body type?

Remember You Are Not Alone

One of the issues in creating a unified theory of weight loss was accounting for the vast number of different types of body shape, behaviours and fitness levels. The advice for someone who has been sedentary and overweight all of their life will be different compared to a professional body builder.

Before you begin your transformation it is helpful to get a general picture of where you are today and to know how many others are in a similar situation as yourself. This is an empowering process as it allows you to see that you are not alone and gives perspective on what you are trying to achieve.

The way to work out how many others are in a similar situation to you is too look at society as a whole.

Body Fat Across the Population

There are different ways to measure body fat, most people use weight as a gauge, including doctors. You can also use clothes size or direct body fat % measurements. All methods have both positives and negatives to them.

Body Mass Index (BMI) By Population

BMI is your weight as an expression of your height. It has been researched extensively as it is the measure adopted by the medical community. To find out your own BMI, divide your weight (kg) by the square of your height in metres. Alternatively, just Google 'BMI calculator' and use one of the free ones that come up.

The graph below shows how BMI varies across the entire population. You can see that the majority of people are either overweight or obese[4].

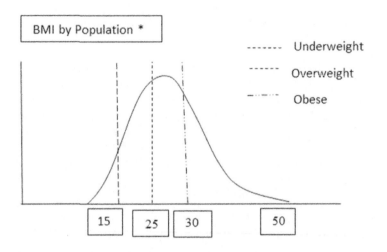

*This is a generalisation for illustration, individual differences exist for age, body type etc.

Body Fat by Population

There are various ways to measure body fat percentage and in general all of the methods can give wildly inaccurate data. This is because they are sensitive to hydrations levels within the body and it is unlikely you will have access to an expensive machine with higher accuracy. With that said the following graph shows what body fat would expect to look like across the population. There are different graphs for Men and Women due to the variations in body fat storage between the sexes. Women have more body fat than men in general due to different physiologies, e.g. breasts. The graph shows that the majority of men and women are considered overweight or obese[5].

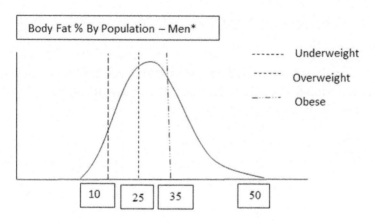

Body Fat % By Population – Men*

------ Underweight
------ Overweight
--·--·- Obese

| 10 | 25 | 35 | | 50 |

*This is a generalisation for illustration, individual differences exist for age, height, body type etc.

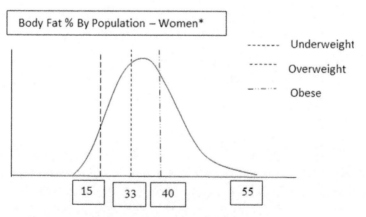

Body Fat % By Population – Women*

------ Underweight
------ Overweight
--·--·- Obese

| 15 | 33 | 40 | | 55 |

*This is a generalisation for illustration, individual differences exist for age, height, body type etc.

Clothes Size by Population

Another classification you can see regularly is clothes size. There is no set standard amongst clothes size as they vary from shop to shop. However, the following graph gives a general insight to clothes size across the overall population.

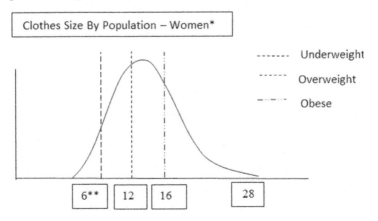

*This is a generalisation for illustration, individual differences exist for age, height, body type etc.

**UK Clothes size

As you can see from the previous graphs, if using medical criteria then the majority of people are overweight these days. Current data for most western countries is that around 60% of people are overweight or obese[6]. This correlates across all body fat measures to therefore give a similar curve on the graphs for BMI, body fat % or clothes size.

As a population in general we are getting larger. This means the curve is shifting to the right alongside our evaluations of what is normal. For example, a normal weight for someone in the 1970's verges on being deemed too thin this day and age, obesity in 1970's was 15% compared to 40% today[7].

Muscle Mass Across the Population

The amount of muscle mass someone has does not have that much measurement data compared to body fat. The vast majority of the population will have average amounts of muscle[8]. While genetic factors exist the predominant influence of how much muscle you have is related to whether you do resistance training. This may be in the form of general life, such as manual work like labouring or formal resistance training like weight lifting. It can also be done in other forms of exercise such as pole dancing, body pump etc.

To have low muscle mass levels your body needs to go through prolonged periods of inactivity or malnourishment. This happens in specific areas of the body when you have an injury or throughout the body if you have are very sedentary life and/or as a result of health conditions that reduce movement. Severe food restriction as seen in people with anorexia will also result in low levels of muscle.

To have high muscle mass you need to do an extended period of resistance training. With less than 20% of the population being a member of a gym[9], it is unlikely anything but a small percentage of people have large amounts of muscle.

The graph on the next page shows the likely distribution of muscle mass within society. As you can see most people have normal ranges of muscle with a small percentage in the low and high muscle mass ends. The very big body builder type physiques associated with gyms are a very tiny percentage of the population.

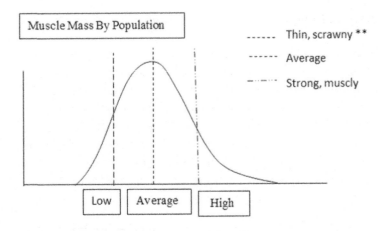

*This is a generalisation for illustration, individual differences exist for age, height, body type etc.

**Typical labels used with these muscle mass levels assuming normal body fat.

***** Questions to Consider *****

-Using the graphs above, where are you currently on the chart for body fat and muscle mass?

-Where would you goal be placed on the previous graphs for body fat and muscle mass?

-How many other people are in the same position as you today? How many other people are at your end goal?

-Who can you identify with based on your goals and current situation?

Drop Your Story

Before you embark on the process of changing your behaviours, thoughts and ultimately your body you will usually need to be open to reviewing the story you tell yourself. We all live by a narrative which is probably not true and it often blocks our progress.

Your story represents what you believe about the world and helps to keep your beliefs consistent. You continually repeat this to yourself and to other people. It influences your thoughts and actions. The key is whether this is helping or hindering your progress.

Any story that closes off your potential for taking action or getting results is not helpful. This may be thinking you are not the type of person who could ever do exercise or that it is impossible to get in shape. It may be a character undermining stories such as you cannot change or you do not have any willpower. It can be entrenched beliefs about your actions that stop you analysing your own behaviours such as 'I barely eat any food' or 'I am very active'. All of these stories can keep you trapped and stop you getting results.

If you are open to dropping your story it simply means you are prepared to listen to the results of taking action. A well designed plan will prove that you are more than what you thought and will allow you to update your self-image and identity. You need to be ok with this type of change and personal growth.

***** Questions to Consider *****

-What stories do you tell yourself that hinder progress?

-What would need to happen to change this narrative?

Accept What Really Creates Change

All too often you assume it is the nutrition or exercise plan that is responsible for transforming your body. This is not true! It is YOU who is responsible for your results. Any plan you use is simply a tool along the journey.

Giving credit to the plan for your results is like saying the bricks, cement and hammer built the house and not the construction workers. The tools and materials will do nothing unless picked up by a motivated and skilled hand that knows what they are doing and then persists until the project is completed.

Getting in shape is the same thing, your nutrition, exercise or movement plans are only as good as your ability to apply them. Results come when you are in the right frame of mind to follow the plans, not because of the plans themselves. Therefore, what will really create change are the actions that put you in this positive and productive mental state.

Longer term, it is the actions that develop your skills and abilities around getting in shape that will determine success. The more skilled you are, the more able you are to adhere to your plans. Therefore the better your results will be.

It is YOU who gets results and thus what truly creates change is the work that helps you grow and develop. You need to focus on what will help unlock your own potential and not obsess over evaluating every detail in a food or exercise plan. You are much more important than any plan or technique.

***** Questions to Consider *****

-How do you currently distribute credit for getting results?

-How would a person vs plan centred approach be different?

Understand How Thoughts, Feelings & Behaviours Can Change

As the key to results is developing your ability to stick to plans and not so much the plans themselves then it is essential you understand the general process to develop these skills.

To adhere to plans better you need to modify how you think, feel and behave going forwards. The fundamental mechanisms by which you can do this are the basis of the Grand Unified Theory of Body Transformations. The following pages describe the main processes, traits and mechanisms by which you can create this change.

This gets very little attention within health and fitness. It is an area that has a lot of potential to be expanded and refined. Hopefully, the future of weight loss will be developed from this angle via psychologists, neuroscientists and behaviour change researchers.

How Behaviours Change Happens

The process behind changing behaviour seems mysterious. Your behaviours can change without any mental focus or even a desire, e.g. you develop bad habits over time. You can of course change your behaviours as millions of people do every year through deciding on how you want to act and then putting a plan in place to change your actions.

There is no set mechanism to changing behaviours like with fat loss or building muscle. This is because there are various inputs and circumstances which act upon a behaviour. This includes whether you are creating a new behaviour or trying to replacing an existing pattern. It also factors in stress amongst others issues.

Though there may not be a set structure there are some core elements within the behaviour change process, including –

Awareness – Becoming conscious of your behaviour patterns is an important element of changing your habits. With no awareness of how you currently act or any better alternatives you will be hard pressed to consciously direct your actions. Your behaviours can change without awareness but this means you are not in control of the process, instead you are subject to the conditions of your environment.

Knowledge – To change behaviours you will often need to acquire new knowledge in or around an area. This may be new information within the process of changing behaviour itself, or related to food or exercise etc. Knowledge can be gained through reading or watching material on the subject but perhaps the best ways to acquire it is by doing the behaviour itself or copying other people's actions.

Skills – Most issues around body transformations need specific skills over knowledge. A skill is achieved through repeated practice of your acquired knowledge. Skills take time to develop and require many repetitions. For example, it is a skill to eat healthily or to exercise when feeling demotivated. Skill and quality practice are inherently related. Likewise, practice and 'failure' go hand in hand while learning a new skill.

Habits & Neural Connection Development – All behaviour change must become automatic for it to be cemented as a long term change. This involves a big element of repetition as well as creation of positive cues and the removal of negative responses towards triggers. This process is the vital link between an awareness and desire to do a new action vs actually being able to do it automatically without thinking.

Emotional Drive –The emotional element of behaviour change cannot be underestimated. The speed that a new behaviour can be formed relates to the number of repetitions verses the emotional intensity experienced. You can change behaviour fairly quickly when emotion is involved. In the absence of it you will need to use a much higher number of repetitions, e.g. how many times did you brush your teeth before it became a habit?

Emotion applies to the desire to change, the feeling experienced upon changing and the emotional responses to cues, triggers and your environment.

Motivation State – This refers to the general emotional state you are experiencing which will determine both how you feel and how you will interpret any given situation. This will influence how you will react to events. For example, if you are in a bad mood you will see neutral events as more negative.

Many behaviour change issues are around changing what motivation states are predominant within your life and/or present in a given environment. The development of a skill usually quietly works on this area as you learn to do the tasks under different states through repeated practice over time.

*****

The behaviour change process does not need to be hard, difficult or unappealing. It can be a fast and fun process depending on how it is done and the attitude taken towards doing it. Any behaviour, including your worst habits can be changed over time with the right approach and a good dose of persistence.

How Feelings / Thoughts Change

In general no one ever gives much consideration on how to change their feelings or thoughts. It is seems to just happen based on what has been going on in life. The normal assumption is that we must achieve something to feel different. This is the underlying belief behind why you or anyone looks to change their body.

While this is a fairly common perspective it is not always true. It is common to see the desired emotional change not accompany physical transformations. This suggests the process of creating new thoughts and feelings is not inherently tied to external changes. So, how do you change how you feel?

In the same way behaviour change does not have a set formula for how it happens, changing your thoughts or feelings likewise does not have a specific set of steps to follow. However, there are various factors that are involved. It is good to understand some of these as they will appear in later sections –

Changing Status Within Your Frame of Reference – Many of your feelings stem from where you have evaluated yourself within your frame of reference of what is good or bad. This is the traditional sense of why you try to achieve a goal, e.g. at dress size 12 you feel bad, dress size 8 you feel amazing. Your feelings have change because of your new evaluation along your current grading scale. If you change your results within your frame you will change how you feel about yourself.

Changing the Frame of Reference – Another way to change how you feel about yourself is to change the frame of evaluation that you are using. We discussed this concept in regards to body positivity which is based on changing what is viewed as a good or bad body shape rather than changing your body within the old set of references. In the previous example, you could change your frame of reference so that you feel good at dress size 12 rather than having to achieve a size 8. The key to this is changing at your subconscious level so you actually feel different rather than wanting or hoping to feel a certain way.

Another element to this is redefining the meaning of what a frame of reference implies about you or others in the world. For example, if you change your beliefs from 'thinner means more attractive' to 'any size can be attractive' it would probably alter the feelings you have around your body.

You do not just have references about your body shape, you have them for your eating behaviours, your career and how you are doing as a person. You probably did not choose most of your frameworks and very often they are not set up to optimise how you feel or the results you achieve in each area.

You can change your frames of reference through looking at the rules, origins and alternatives to your current structures.

Changing the Emotional Perspective System - In the great book, 'How Emotions Are Made' by Lisa Feidman Barrett, she discusses how the brain creates an emotional prediction before you experience the actual emotion. This means that you can change how you feel by changing the predictive system. This can be influenced by various subconscious elements including physiology, e.g. the warm mug experiment where the holder perceives a situation more positively when given a warm drink to hold compared to a cold one[10].

She also discusses emotional granulation, which is looking at the different types of emotions you perceive. This involves being able to identify and differentiate between more of the emotions that you experience. The greater your repertoire of emotion the larger your potential to change how you feel. Through practice you can expand your emotional vocabulary.

Dissociating Emotions From a Thought / Memory – It may be that the way to change your feelings in the current moment is to dissociate from an emotion attached to a particular thought or memory from the past. This can be done using various techniques, some of which we will discuss later.

When the emotion is no longer attached to the thoughts or memory you will feel different in the present day. This may be the stimulus needed to create change within your life.

Knowledge – Learning new things, sometimes factually, but very often from a self-perspective and self-learning sense can be enough to change how you perceive yourself or perceive an issue. This could mean you reclassify yourself within a frame of reference or change the meaning or grade of the reference itself and therefore how you feel.

Questioning the Assumptions of Your Thoughts – Your thought process can be changed by asking about and revealing the hidden assumptions, meanings and basis upon which they may exist. This investigation can be done via the use of metaphor or direct questioning.

Associating With People – The Influence of Others – Change often only happens via the influence of other people, this could be within a formal coaching process or just by being around people with different behaviours or beliefs. Along similar lines, sometimes you will be unable to change how you feel while still in the prescience of other people. Especially if they strongly hold beliefs you are trying to get away from.

Repetition & Association – The base process behind changing how you feel about doing tasks is through repetition. The same applies in learning to think differently or more positively, you will need to repeat it many times for it to become a natural way of being. Over time great changes can happen through this simple process.

*****

So what does this look like in practice?

To change your feelings around a small trait like not enjoying exercise you may need to first question and change your beliefs around not being the kind of person who is ever active. Then you may need to remind yourself of any positive experiences of exercising that you have had. With this done you are ready to start with a very small, short and fun exercise routine to gradually develop positive feelings around movement. You would then build upon this over time by using friends or fitness professionals to teach you more around exercise.

In a bigger issue such as improving confidence you may need to investigate various frames of references behind why you do not feel confident currently. You may need to also address some previous emotional events which underpin the problem. In addition to this you could start doing behaviours which make you feel confident today and gradually condition this feeling into your body over time. You would also want to increase the interactions with other people who develop your confidence and reduce your contact with those who diminish this feeling.

Summary Section 1

-**Change is Possible** – You need to believe in the possibility you could change. Actions create change and there is nothing to stop you being successful if you do the right actions. You can achieve your goals! Believe in the possibility of your success, even if it just from a position of hope.

-**YOU Are Not Your Body or Your Behaviours** – You need to learn to manage and work with your body and behaviours as you are not completely in control of them. The goal is to have all three elements in alignment moving forwards.

-**The Three Body Transformation Lies** – Do not fall for these common misconceptions. Changing your body is not about knowledge, effort or motivation. It is about developing skills, sticking to it for the duration and being persistent. Every transformation is a unique challenge based off your whole history. So avoid thinking it should be easy for you because someone else appears to do it effortlessly and be careful of expecting other plans to work for you without first tailoring them to your needs.

-**Balance The Traditional Goal Vs Body Positivity Approach** – Either extreme can cause problems and prevent progress. You should like who you are and where you are today but be excited and inspired to progress and change your body.

-**Your Feelings About Change** – Half the population do not like change or only get motivated when there is a problem they need to get away from. If this is you then spend time thinking about how you are heading in a direction you do not want to be going and how you must change now to avoid this fate.

-**Body Shape Influences** – How you look has many factors, the ones you can significantly change are body fat, muscle mass and posture. Other factors such as height, body fat distribution pattern and facial features are hard or impossible to change. You should focus only on the things that can change and work on accepting the elements that cannot.

-**Body Shape Across The Population** – The majority of the population are overweight and have low to average muscle mass. There is a good chance your body is not as bad as you think it is and is actually fairly common along the population spectrum. Be wary of comparing yourself to fitness models on magazines who are the top 0.1% of all people.

-**Be Open to Change** – The harder and more forcefully you try to hold onto your current beliefs and personal story the harder change will become. Ensure you are open to possibility and seeing the reactions of any plans you try.

-**Results Come From Behaviour Change** – Short term success comes from any action that puts you in the right frame of mind to follow your plans better. Longer term results come from actions that develop your skills so you can stick to your plans more easily. Avoid getting distracted by different diet or exercise plans. They are the tools used by you. They are only as effective as your current level of skills and general mental outlook. Plans are meaningless if you cannot follow them.

-**Changing Behaviours, Thoughts & Feelings** – There is no set standard approach to creating new behaviours or thinking processes. There are various elements that may or may not go into it which depends on your history and the make-up of what you are trying to change.

****

Richard, 58 – A successful lawyer, he has a crazy workload managing his team and attending cases. He has never done formal exercise, instead only playing tennis and golf which he does much less frequently now. His weight has increased over the last 10 years and he has various aches and pains on his body. He eats out a lot and drinks regularly. On weekends he usually goes out for dinner with his wife/friends.

A conventional approach would be for Richard to get a Personal Trainer. He would see him twice a week, work hard but within his limits and be told to be more sensible with his food and drink. He would progress initially with his fitness but eventually become inconsistent and stall. Ultimately he would achieve few results and soon be back to square one.

Richard came to me for personal training but agreed to change his focus to give health & fitness equal priority when making his diary. He planned in time to walk and we recorded his steps. We trained together once a week but on top of this he agreed to do a behaviour change programme to consciously choose whether he wanted to eat or drink while out. This involved a series of mini experiments where he purposefully altered just one element of his behaviour, e.g. at lunch he would not have wine or no starter for dinner etc.

Using this approach Richard was able to break the numerous automatic 'bad' behaviours he was doing. No longer did he open a bottle of wine the moment he walked in the door, he would now decide if he wanted it or not. At a restaurant he would ask himself if he was hungry before ordering a desert. He still did his 'bad' behaviours but now that he was more active and conscious with his decisions things were different. He managed to lose 15kg and sustain it.

****

The Grand Unified Theory of Weight Loss

Section 2

The Mechanics of Physical Change

All you need to know about changing your body is outlined here in this section. You will learn exactly what is needed to be done to lose every bit of body fat to get to your goal or add significant amounts of muscle up to that of a bodybuilder if you so desire.

You will also learn about how to change your posture, flatten your stomach and achieve other holistic elements such as getting fitter and improving your health.

This section focuses only on the physical actions you need to take. It rests on the assumption you can follow exactly what you are meant to do. This assumption is total lunacy of course. If you could do exactly what you wanted to do you would have achieved all of your goals a long time ago.

The rest of the book after this section will look at how to get you to do these needed actions. This is done by using various behaviour change strategies to create habits and new sustainable behaviours patterns.

It is important and very helpful to understand the true mechanism by which you can change your body and the subtle changes that are needed for continued results. Most people are lacking this knowledge which makes it harder to get to your goals. This is especially true if you have struggled to lose weight before or if you have big goals in terms of how much you want to change your body.

How Do You Lose Fat

It is beyond vital you get a firm and sensible understanding of how to lose fat. The process of losing fat/weight has reached almost mystical proportions with all sorts of crazy theories confusing people left, right and centre.

The following chapters detail the process around how you lose fat. Your thoughts on this are probably clouded due to information overload from your previous efforts. Therefore, this is the time to learn what knowledge to keep and what to discard.

The following pages give you the practical and functional knowledge to get results. There is a very simplistic model and a more in-depth version. The simple version is good enough for results alongside a behaviour change plan. The more in-depth version makes any transformation a little easier. Either way, real world transformations come from changing behaviours and developing skills and not in-depth biochemistry knowledge.

Please note that losing weight, toning up, slimming down are all terms describing fat loss. For most people the terms weight loss and fat loss are interchangeable.

The Super Basic View of How to Lose Fat

Body fat is an energy store which can be used if food supplies run short. It also fulfils various other purposes within the body and we need it to be healthy. If you consume too much food over a prolonged period of time you will accumulate fat. At a certain threshold of gained additional fat you will feel you want to lose 'weight' (body fat).

The determining factor for fat loss is your energy balance. This can be measured in calories. While factors affect energy consumed and expended as discussed below, the ultimate determinant of fat loss is energy in vs energy out.

If you take anyone and lock them away in a prison cell while feeding them a very low calorie diet they will lose fat every time. The problem is that you are not locked away in a cell but you live in the free world where food is everywhere.

Your energy balance can be summed up by:

ENERGY BALANCE = FOOD INTAKE − ENERGY NEEDED

So if you eat 2000 calories in a day but expend 3000 you will have an energy balance of -1000 calories, which will produce fat loss. Alternatively, if you eat 3000 calories but expend only 2000 you will have +1000 calories energy balance, which will produce fat gain.

There can be daily variations to the calorie balance equations so it can be better to look at it over a week, e.g. you needed 21000 calories but ate 14000 so you have lost body fat.

How many calories you need is summed up by:

CALORIE NEEDS = YOUR BODY'S BASIC CALORIFIC NEEDS TO FUNCTION + MOVEMENT IN LIFE (EXERCISE+WALKING)

This could mean your basic calorie needs are 1500 calories, plus 300 calories from walking and 200 calories from exercise. This would give a total of 2000 calories needed for that day. In weekly terms this means you need 14 000 calories. If you were to eat over that amount you will gain fat, if you eat under that amount you will lose fat. The greater the calorie excess or deficit you consume, the larger the change in body fat in either direction.

Exercise and movement are interchangeable when it comes to fat loss. You can get results through simply walking or via exercise which may be long and steady cardio, high intensity sessions or resistance training. None of these are the 'best' way to exercise. It is just about how you balance it with your food intake for results.

A significant percentage of the population will eat more food when they exercise than when they do not[11]. If this is you then walking would be a better method for losing body fat than formal more challenging exercise. This is because you may be unable to control your hunger after your fitness session and therefore accidently end up eating more food than you burnt during the session itself.

The biggest influence on fat loss at a practical level is usually your food intake. The nature of high calorie food is that you can eat in minutes what it takes to burn off in hours. Foods vary greatly in how many calories they contain and you need to balance energy content with taste and enjoyment.

****

The above equations are at the heart of the fat loss process. Too often people deny this mechanism and look for more complicated solutions. You can quite easily use this super simplistic model as your base to get results and lose weight alongside an effective behaviour management process.

The Practical View of How to Lose Fat

So we know that energy balance determines what happens to your body fat. If you want to lose it then you need to eat less than you expend over a week or a month. It is helpful to take this knowledge a little deeper and look at some other factors and facets of fat loss that have practical implications. This includes basic nutrition, biology and various fat loss myths.

The Structure of 'Body Fat' & It's Misleading Name

A slightly unhelpful and confusing element in all this is the term body fat. The fat that you can grab is called adipose tissue and it contains our reserve energy stores. It is not an inert tissue but rather it plays an important role within the body producing hormones, influencing hunger and storing toxins amongst other functions[12].

Within the adipose tissue there are 'empty' containers that will fill up if you consume more energy than you expend. It is the filling up or emptying of these containers that causes you to gain or lose 'weight'. The containers are filled up with a molecule that combines one carbohydrate (called glycerol) with three chains of fat[13]. Therefore, instead of calling our excess weight 'fat', we should call it 'carbo-fat' or similar.

Your body has ways to create this molecule and therefore store fat if you overeat on protein, carbohydrates or fat. It is not the type of food that determines fat gain but the overall amount you consume. To empty the containers you will need to use up the molecules which will depend on your energy balance. It is not related to whether you eat a diet low in fat or carbohydrates. Any reference to losing or gaining 'body fat' is referring to changes in these carbo-fat energy reserves.

Energy Explained

Your energy balance determines how you change appearance. Energy is measured by calories. Officially, 1 calorie is the amount of energy it takes to raise 1 litre of water by $1c^{14}$. In real terms it is the most specific way to measure how much food you have eaten or see the amount of energy expended by moving or exercising.

There are all sorts of issues with calories that people complain about. This includes how badly most people measure them, the different effects certain calorie types have on the body and the difficulty estimating calories burnt in exercise.

However, despite some very valid criticisms there is still no better method out there for determining the amount of food eaten or energy expended.

What Influences How Many Calories Your Body Needs?

It only makes sense if looking to manipulate the energy balance equation to want to know how to increase the calories you are burning. There are various factors that affect how many calories you burn per day, some can be changed while others cannot. The following affect how many calories you need but generally are not that easy to manipulate:

Size – How big a bodied person you are in general will influence how many calories you need, e.g. a tall large framed man will burn more calories than a short petite woman.

Weight –You burn more calories when you are heavier simply from moving more weight around. The same would apply if you were carrying a heavy backpack. As you lose weight during a transformation you will expend less energy than before for the same amount of movement as you are lighter.

Metabolism –The strength of your metabolism represents various biochemical processes going on within the body. This includes cell regeneration, detoxification and your internal body temperature. The thyroid gland's efficiency influences this process to some degree. Metabolism varies across the population and even between people of the same size.

Temperature –The climate you are exposed affects calorie burn, e.g. you would burn more calories if you work outside during the winter as you try to keep warm than working inside an office with heating.

Body Position – You will burn more calories standing up than sitting down and even less calories lying down.

Mental Engagement – Your brain activity affects calorie usage. You will burn more calories when trying to solve a difficult problem than when you are watching TV. You expend the least calories when you are asleep.

Monthly Cycle – Women will experience variations during their monthly cycle for how many calories they need per day. This can range from 50-200+ calories per day difference.

Medications & Supplements – Many medications affect your metabolism, some can increase your calorie needs while many reduce it. Some supplements have the same effect.

Involuntary Movements – Fidgeting, which is mostly involuntary can burn extra calories. It is often used by the body to expend excess calories consumed.

Nutrition – What, How Much & How Often You Eat – The types of food you consume affect the energy burn of the body. Likewise, the more times you eat per day the more calories you burn if the amount of food is kept constant. This is due to the energy cost of digestion.

However, you need to be careful with this aspect. Doubling the amount of food you eat to burn 50 extra calories digesting it is not a good idea. Your recent nutrition will also affect your metabolism, long periods of under eating decreases your metabolism and long periods of overeating increases it.

Temperature of Liquids Consumed – Very cold liquids when consumed use energy to raise your body temperature. For most this is impractical to be able to generate much in terms of energy demands, however, it is a factor on overall intake.

*****

In reality it is not so easy to change many of the above elements. You could stand up at work more, lower the office temperature and not wear a jumper but then you may find your work performance suffers because you are not comfortable and feel cold. You could walk everywhere carrying a 10kg weight vest, drink 3 litres of ice cold water a day or leave a note to fidget more. All of this is much harder to do in comparison to just doing the obvious ways to burn more calories which are:

Exercise – Doing exercise uses energy, the longer you do it the more calories you burn. In general aerobic exercise burns more calories than resistance. Harder exercise burns more calories per minute than easier exercise but you need to consider how many minutes of each you can do.

Exercise - EPOC – While calories are burnt when exercising you also burn extra energy following an exercise session. A hard exercise session can increase your calorie burn for the next 24 hours[15]. In general, the harder the exercise, the greater the extra energy expenditure will be after the session. It is best to view the exercise session and EPOC together for a fair evaluation of the overall calorie burn when comparing different exercise types.

Movement – This refers to how much you move about in life, e.g. walking steps, gentle cycling to work etc. This can come from a focused effort like going for a walk or as a natural consequence of your lifestyle, e.g. a postman would walk much further than an office worker in a typical day. Low level movements such as walking or cycling offer a huge calorie burn opportunity as you can walk large distances if you have the time without injury.

Activities – Any activity that engages your brain, involves movement or gets you up on your feet will burn more calories than the nations favourite activities of watching TV or surfing the net. Almost any hobby would come under this category.

Relative Energy Contributions

The majority of your calorie needs stem from the base processes within your body. This includes the energy used per day just to exist and the calories used in the digestion process. This can vary based on the factors discussed already.

For most people these base processes account for 75-90% of your calorie needs. So if you need 2000 calories a day, 1600 may come just from your body's needs. This means that your movement and exercise is relatively a small contributor for most people, especially if you have a sedentary lifestyle.

If you increased your steps or added in a big workout you can greatly increase your calorie needs albeit the base processes will still usually be the biggest energy user. For example, in the previous case, adding in 500 calories of movement or exercise would mean your total needs are 2500 calories a day, where 1600 calories are from your base needs and 900 from movement.

This is important to understand as it shows that exercise or movement is not some magical saviour but rather it nudges the energy balance in your favour. It also shows why steps and movement in life are so important. It is hard to expend a lot of energy through exercise alone because you get tired and it takes motivation and time dedicated to it.

However, steps represent a huge potential to increase energy burn without much effort and they can be integrated into your general life. This means you do not need to beat yourself up about exercise when you could just move more in other ways. You can see the relative energy contributions of the base processes of the body vs movement & exercise within your total energy needs in the chart below.

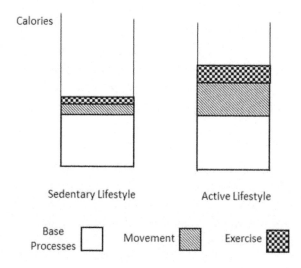

While exercise and movement increase your overall energy needs this will usually not produce significant changes in body fat unless you also address your food alongside it.

Calories Within Food

The other side to the energy balance equation is calorie intake. There is not a set amount of calories within food as it depends upon what the food is made up from and how much of it you eat. This can vary greatly between meals. Any food will contain one or more of the following –

Food	Calories / Gram	Notes
Protein	4	Macro Nutrients
Carbohydrates	4	
Fat	9	
Alcohol	7	
Water	0	
Vitamins	0	Micro Nutrients
Minerals	0	

How many calories a food contains comes back to the proportions of the protein, carbs and fat within it. For the purposes of this discussion I will not include alcohol within foods as it is mostly only found in alcoholic drinks.

Food Density

At a practical level it is important to understand the issue of food density. Each individual food has its own percentages of water, protein, carbs and fat. The less water the higher the energy density. The major component of most foods is water. For example take a look at this list of foods[16]:

Food	% Water	% Protein	% Carbs	% Fat	Cals/100g
Lettuce	97%	1%	3%	0%	16
Carrot	91%	1%	8%	0%	36
Bananas	76%	1%	23%	0%	96
Tuna	74%	25%	0%	1%	109
Rice	69%	3%	28%	0%	124
Pasta	69%	5%	25%	1%	129
Chicken breast	68%	29%	0%	3%	143
Olive Oil	0%	0%	0%	100%	900

As you can see, the different foods have varying nutrient amounts within them. Vegetables are over 95% water while olive oil is 100% fat. Some foods have protein, carbs and fat while others have just one of these.

This means the same amount of food will have greatly different calorie intake. 100 grams of chocolate has around 530 calories while 100g of green vegetables has just 25 calories. You would therefore need different amounts of food on your plate to provide the same amount of energy. For example, to consume 50 grams of carbohydrates (~200 calories) you would need to eat just under 200g of cooked rice or over 600 grams of carrots. Most people would struggle to eat that amount of carrots.

It is for this reason many diets suggest eating vegetables due to their low energy density. It means you can eat a lot of veg yet will not consume that many calories. Conversely junk food is criticised due to the high energy density as you will not need to eat much to consume a lot of calories.

However, your energy consumption comes back to how many calories you eat. There is nothing wrong with eating any food as long as the amount of energy consumed is considered.

What Influences How Many Calories You Consume?

How much food you actually eat in the real world is influenced by many different elements. You probably do most of your eating while on automatic therefore you will be influenced by one or more of the following;

Frequency of Eating – As a society we eat more often than we ever have before. You may find yourself eating every two to three hours, you will snack on the way home before dinner and often straight afterwards. It is not necessarily bad to eat frequently but the more often you eat the easier it is to consume more calories.

Food Density – The modern day diet is characterised by very high calorie dense foods. This means you can eat what may appear like almost nothing e.g. a handful of nuts or a few biscuits, but it has the same calories as a small meal. The foods within our diet are becoming more calorific with less emphasis on lower calorie dense foods such as vegetables. This makes it easy to eat more and overeat.

Exercise Compensation – As mentioned previously a certain percentage of the population are known as exercise compensators[18]. This means that they may burn 300 calories by doing exercise but will have a natural tendency to eat more calories than this after the session. This could mean that despite your best exercise efforts you are accidently increasing hunger and food intake simultaneously.

Habitual Behaviours – The vast majority of your eating happens while you are on automatic and without even thinking about it. This includes how you respond to food cues, your reaction to certain types of taste and the influence of other people on your behaviours.

Hunger – The hungrier you are the more likely you are to eat more food. As a society we have become very out of touch with our natural hunger patterns or knowing when we are full. We also often fear the feeling of hunger and grab something to eat at the very first sensation of it. There are different causes of hunger and the body can be developed to be more or less hungry over time.

Emotions / Stress – The more stressed you are the more likely you are to eat too much food. Eating food is the easiest and most available way to try to satisfy stress even though it is very ineffective at actually fighting against it. You may also eat when you are experiencing different emotions such as when you are bored or if you are feeling sad.

*****

There are other factors alongside the above ones but this gives you an insight into some of your drivers to eat. Just using these traits alone you could easily reduce food intake.

If you were to eat slightly less often with lower calorie dense foods it would be a great start. If you examined your hunger and exercise relationship and matched your movement to fit that would also help. Likewise, any work on reconnecting to a more natural hunger – fullness pattern, or becoming conscious when eating would reduce food intake as well.

Macro Nutrients – Protein, Carbs & Fat

The issue of 'macros' has been very popular in recent years around body transformations. Macros refer to the main calorie providers of protein, carbs and fat. This is opposed to micro nutrients which are your vitamins and minerals.

Macros as an Energy Source

Usually your energy will be supplied predominantly from fat and carbohydrates with just a little from protein[17]. The ratios of fat and carbs used will change when you do exercise depending on the type and duration of it.

The body has the ability to change which macros it uses for energy burning. For example, if you go low carb the body will up-regulate your fat usage and vice versa, if you eat high carb, you will use more carbohydrates for energy at rest. High protein intake will also up-regulate protein energy utilisation. There are individual differences in the ideal macro ratio and it is possible for this ideal ratio to change at different points during your life.

Macros & Fat Loss

The balance of macro energy usage does not influence how much body fat you lose. The most important element for fat loss is whether you create a calorie deficit. With any practical eating plan your results will be directly related to the size of your calorie deficit regardless of what macro ratio you use.

There are some interesting debates on how changes in a macro group could affect the body, e.g. what if you only eat protein or never eat any fat. This also include issues of calorie intake, e.g. if you lose body fat on 1800 calories a day can you get the same results adding an extra 200 calories of protein.

While these are fun debates they are unnecessary at a practical level. Almost no one eliminates whole macro groups for extended periods of time and for the vast majority of people their diets are surprisingly consistent across a week.

Your macros will be roughly similar for all of your 'good' days and all of your 'bad' days, though they will often be different between 'good' vs 'bad' days. This means in the real world you need to focus on your energy balance as the primary mechanism to change your body.

Where Macros Really Help

The ratio of protein to carbs to fat has a significant effect on satiety levels, cravings and how you feel following a meal. It also affects the total amount of food you need to eat in a day to feel satisfied.

When you eat with the right ratio for your body you should be without hunger, cravings or the desire to eat for the next few hours. You will also experience good mental and physical energy.

If you eat with the wrong ratio you may feel hunger within two hours of eating even if you 'feel full'. Your energy could drop and your mental focus may be off.

The same applies per day, if you eat with the right ratio for your body you can be full and satisfied on much lower overall amounts of food than with the wrong ratio.

The ideal macro ratio varies, for some people it could be 20% protein and 60% carbs while others 40% protein and 30% carbs. You must find what works for you. In general, you will probably not do well when any macro group is very low or eliminated. Most people need all three in some form.

The average person's diet this day and age is usually too low in protein to optimise post meal reactions. It is common to see protein intake at around 5-15% of total energy intake. If this is you then I would expect you to feel more satisfied by adding a little more protein into your diet in some form.

The Six Types of Hunger

There is a direct correlation between hunger and how much you eat. To reduce food intake you will need to understand the various types of hunger and how they are addressed differently. It is common to blame yourself for being weak willed around food when you are actually just not fulfilling the needs of the different hungers. The main hunger types are:

Normal Hunger – This is a natural and calm desire for food. The hunger builds gradually and evenly while coming and going in waves. You can usually resist it fairly easily until it rises to a high level. This natural feeling should be listened to. This hunger will always be present throughout your life and should be satisfied when it arises. When this is the only type of hunger you experience you will feel calm when eating and have an easy relationship with food.

Water Hunger – A thirst for water is like normal hunger in that it usually grows gradually and evenly. It is a fairly calm request on the body that you can easily manage. However, if you always eat food instead of drinking you may find yourself continually eating and not understanding why. A water hunger can occur without you actually feeling thirsty if you keep eating as it masks the thirst feeling.

This issue is easily countered by drinking water regularly throughout the day. Note, for some people drinking too much water can cause a low blood sugar hunger as detailed below which therefore increase the amount of hunger experienced.

You goal is to drink adequate amounts of water for your body, not too much or too little. How often you go to the toilet will give you a clue if you are drinking the right amount as well as the volume and colour of your urine.

Macro's Hunger – This is one of the most common causes of hunger and perhaps the biggest reason people wrongly blame their eating on emotions. It comes from inefficient energy production and/or inadequate signals from within your digestive system. As discussed this happens after you eat a meal with the incorrect ratio or amount of Protein: Carbohydrates: Fat for your body. It can cause you to get a hunger feeling, often in the form of a sugar craving, anywhere from 15 minutes up to 3 hours after eating.

This is usually the reason that you can find yourself hungry fairly soon after having a meal despite the fact you "should" be full. The way to counter this is to eat each meal with the correct macro ratio for your body. This can be found out through experimentation and listening to the body's reactions after eating.

Blood Sugar Hunger –This is a powerful hunger. When your blood sugar levels drop below a certain value your hormone system kicks in to regulate your metabolism. This puts an unwelcome stress on your body long term and in the short term can produce some very strong food cravings and hunger. The onset can be fast and it will cause a sugar craving.

Low blood sugar problems can be resolved in the short term by eating regularly and ensuring you are eating in accordance to your ideal macro ratio. Drinking too much water can also reduce your blood sugar which could cause you to eat more. Experimentation can reveal the ideal amount for you.

Blood sugar metabolism is a sign of many different factors and processes. Therefore, long term resolution of high or low blood sugar problems comes from addressing your body's overall functioning and health.

Brain Based Hunger – This refers to a craving or hunger that stems from your brain. There are different possible underlying causes to this. It could be neurotransmitter imbalances or through the dopamine/food reward pathway. Habitual based behavioural cravings would come under this category also, e.g. you crave popcorn because you are at the cinema. It has been suggested that cravings can arise from low glycogen levels in the liver or deficiencies in certain vitamins / minerals in the body. The evidence is not quite so clear if this is true but if it then it would activate this desire through mechanisms in the brain.

Regardless of the source, a brain based hunger usually operates independently to natural hunger or nutritional needs. This type of hunger is almost always mistakenly viewed as an emotional hunger. You can resolve this issue through experimenting with the different underlying causes.

Emotional Hunger – True emotional hunger has nothing to do with nutritional cravings. An emotional craving has a very fast onset, often instantaneously. For example, you receive a phone call that makes you angry and immediately you are snacking on some biscuits. Maybe you speak to someone about money and straightaway you are having a piece of cake. You may do this without even thinking or noticing yourself doing it. These cravings can come and go very quickly.

The emotional cause of your poor eating may be obvious, e.g. just broke up with your partner, or more subtle stemming from the stress of your current life situation. This area is best addressed through using stress management techniques in the short term and changing how you respond to emotions in the long term.

Interplay of the Different Types of Hunger

All the hungers have the potential to act upon you and you should learn how to handle them. To begin this process you could try eating regularly with the right macro ratios while drinking adequate amounts of water. This would form a good base to explore the other types of hunger.

The Wavelike Nature of Hunger

When dealing with all of the hunger types they usually come in waves. This means you do not battle hunger all day long but you will feel a hunger sensation for a short period of time (5-20 minutes) which will then disappear and come back later. This may be 30 minutes or many hours afterwards.

The problem for most people is they eat at the first sensation of hunger. Assuming you have taken a fairly sensible approach with your base eating regime there is nothing wrong with sitting through gentle hunger and waiting for it to disappear. The body is clever, if it needs something it will ask you fairly soon afterwards to go and eat. However, in the vast majority of cases you will find that the hunger signal was 'fake news'.

Reconnecting to Natural Hunger-Fullness Patterns

The body is adaptable. If you eat every couple of hours it will expect to be fed frequently and vice versa, if you go for periods without eating your body will become comfortable not eating. Historically, our bodies were designed to handle temporary food shortages from back when our supplies were less reliable. Even though we may be designed to go without food it is common to need to retrain your brain/body to go be comfortable not eating. With a little practice and focus it is possible to restore a more natural hunger–fullness pattern.

Hunger Hormones

Two elements involved with some of hunger processes[19] outlined above are Ghrelin, the hormone that makes you hungry and Leptin, the hormone that reduces appetite. In many people these can become dis-regulated and out of balance which will influence your hunger and eating patterns.

You can look to improve how these hunger hormones interact within your body by examining your macro ratios and seeing which eating patterns fill you up the most. This varies between individuals. The next thing you can do is address your sleep as it influences hormone regulation.

Taste

The absence of taste within your eating can increase hunger and the amount of food consumed. A low level of taste is one of the main reasons you will quit your plan. The issue with taste is how to increase it without significantly raising the quantity of food you eat per day.

There are different properties of taste, e.g. saltiness, firmness sweetness, temperature. What you like the most is individual to you but also varies with your mood. For example, you may prefer spicier food yet some days you will want a sweeter taste over spicy one for dinner. You can train your body to like an element of taste and also change how much food you need to satisfy a specific element.

If you are aware of the property of taste you want to eat you can use it to make lower calorie choices while also meeting your taste needs, e.g. if you want something cold you could choose an ice lolly over ice cream, if want something crunchy you could have frozen berries over nuts or if looking for warmth you could make your salad into a warm soup.

The Energy Balance Equation – 1 Day vs 7 Day Variation

You know how to burn more calories and can see some of the base principles behind eating less. This means you can apply both of these to create an energy deficit and therefore force the body to fill the gap by tapping into your fat stores.

In the simplistic view of fat loss discussed previously it was assumed that if you under eat by 1 calorie you would lose 1 calorie of body fat and vice versa if you overate. The same would apply for 100 or 1000 calories.

While this is fairly true in a long term sense it is not actually true in a short term sense, especially over a 24 hour period. This is important because it gives more freedom to your routine and explains some of the quirks of fat loss.

To explain this concept you need to understand more about your energy reserves in the body and the body's ability to vary its metabolic processes.

Energy Reserves

As you already know, body fat represents a reserve energy store. However, it is not the only source available. You have both carbohydrates and protein as well. Your carbohydrates are stored in the muscles or your liver. If needed the body can also break down your muscle to liberate protein and create energy. On top of this there is the fat, carbs and protein entering the system from your meals. The table below sums up some of the main features of each energy reserve[20].

Energy Store	Location	Energy/Kg	Energy Store*	Ease of Access
Body Fat	Around the body	7700 cals	50 000 cals+	Easy
Carbs	Muscles, Liver	4100 cals	2-5000 cals+	Easy - Medium
Protein	Muscles	4200 cals	30 000 cals+	Hard
*Stores vary depending on excess body fat levels and amount of muscle tissue				

So the energy balance equation now needs to consider what will happen in the body if you overeat or under eat.

In an ideal world if you ate 100 calories less than you need your body would tap into your body fat stores and you would be a little thinner as a result. However, it does not have to do this, the body could tap into the carb sources in your liver to fill the energy deficit. This would mean you are no thinner despite under eating by 100 calories ☹

It is not all doom and gloom though as this can go the other way too. You could overeat by a 100 calories and your body could handle the excess energy by storing it as carbohydrates. So you have eaten 100 calories too much yet have not gained any body fat ☺

Your Body's Ability to Vary Metabolic Processes

The other side to the energy balance issue is what the body chooses to do with its metabolism when you eat too much or too little.

If we continue the 100 calorie example, it could be that you have under eaten by 100 calories and in response to this your body slows down your metabolic process so you actually need 100 calories less that day than you thought. You did everything right but you have not lost body fat ☹

The flipside to this is that you overeat by 100 calories and your body responds by raising your metabolic rate to use up the excess 100 calories. So you messed up and ate too much yet you did not gain any body fat ☺

So What Happens in Reality if You Under Eat Today? - There is no definite way to know if your body will tap into your body fat stores to make up the calorie deficit or instead use your carb stores or reduce your metabolic rate. How the body chooses to responds today is influenced by the size of the deficit, types of foods consumed, your previous behaviours before today and has a genetic element to it.

So What Happens if You Under Eat for a Whole Week? This is a little easier to answer, the body will mobilise your body fat to make up some of the deficit. This is because the more the carbohydrate reserves are depleted the less likely the body is to want to use them for filling the energy deficit. Therefore we know you will start tapping into your body fat. Likewise, while the body may drop its metabolic rate initially it will soon stabilise at the new level even if you are under eating. This may mean your predicted fat loss is less than the initial numbers predicted but you will still be losing body fat.

So What Happens in Reality if I Over Eat Today? – The body could respond by storing the excess carbohydrates and using the fat you ate as fuel or by increasing your metabolic rate to use more of the excess energy. Alternatively you could store the excess calories as body fat. You do not know how your body will respond as it is varies between people. Studies have shown that the type of foods you eat can influence how much of it you store alongside other factors such as previous nutrition and the size of the calorie surplus[21].

What Happens if I Over Eat for a Whole Week? – This is again easier to answer, before long your carb stores will be full and there will be an excess of carbs and fats in the system. Your body will become stable in how much it will raise your metabolic rate and at that point you will begin to store excess calories as body fat.

As you can see, when looked at over a seven day period or longer the body will gain or lose body fat based on your energy balance.

The subtle differences that happen over a 24 hour period are important to understand because it means you can drop your attachment to having a specific calorie number by which your life is ruled. You do not gain body fat the moment you eat over your daily calorie number. You cannot be that accurate with the calories in / out model. In this sense it is maybe better to look at your calorie needs as a weekly number, e.g. 14000 per week not 2000 per day.

The fact only long term overeating causes body fat gain is encouraging as if you have 1 or 2 bad days there is a good chance you have not gained any body fat yet. This means you can regroup and start again.

Food Absorption

The calories model of fat loss usually assumes that you absorb all of the food that you eat. This is not true in the real world and how much food you do absorb will vary between you and the next person and whether you eat too much or too little.

Studies have shown a significant variety in absorption rates between individuals under different eating conditions[22]. This adds further reasons to why you should not get fixated on short term eating evaluations and calorie amounts.

The amount of calories you eat that are actually absorbed will be part of the reason why some people find it easier to lose or maintain their body weight than others. It will also contribute to the big differences seen in food intake requirements amongst similar sized individuals.

The Fat Loss Behaviour Test

An important evaluation of your skills around changing your body is whether you have the ability to lose fat simply through walking and controlling your food. You need to be able to do this. Losing body fat by monitoring your steps and adjusting your food to create a calorie deficit is the fundamental base of fat loss.

When you are able to do this you can discard all the crazy theories about what you need to do to lose weight. This is the practical way to truly understand fat loss. For most people though they will need to work on a few of the behaviour aspects identified in section 3 to be able to follow this option.

This approach is good in regards to perceived effort. One of the problems with hard-core efforts of extreme exercise plans or strict diets is that they can stop you following them again in the future. This is because you remember the negative and difficult elements of the extreme approach. Fat loss by walking with a sensible calorie deficit is very low effort and will create few negative associations.

Through doing this test you will also be able to see if you are an exercise compensator, that is, someone who will naturally eat more as a result of exercising. If this applies to you then the walking fat loss test will be a surprise in how easy it is to actually get results.

An inability to be able to lose body fat this way shows you have more to develop around your eating behaviours or movement patterns.

The way to monitor you walking is by counting steps. Almost every phone has a step counter on it these days or you can download a free app to count them. You can also buy various wrist step counters.

There are no rights or wrongs about how many steps you should move per day. The less you move the better your food needs to be and vice versa. Food adherence refers primarily to quantity and intake amount over the types of food. You need to find the right balance for you to lose fat. As a guide:

7 Day Step Average	Food Quantity (Calories*)	Food Adherence Level
<5000	Very Low	Amazing
5000-8000	Low	Very good
8000-12000	Low to Medium	Good
12000-18000	Medium	Average to Good
18000+	Medium to high	Average
*Always personalise food intake or calorie amounts to your own needs.		

The steps can be slow and gentle. You are not doing fitness work. Longer term you can exercise obviously and there are many unique health benefits from doing it. However, fat loss is built on this simple foundation of movement vs food.

Steps offer an almost unlimited potential to increase energy use safely. If you were to jog 10000 steps (~7km) every day you would soon get injured. However, you could easily walk 20 000 steps (~14km) every day for a year. The main issue is time it takes to do it. You roughly walk at 6000 steps per hour. The calorie demand of walking vs your weight is below[23]:

Energy Demand of Steps (Calories) vs Body Weight*			
Steps	60kg	80kg	100kg
5000 (3.5km)	170	230	286
7500 (5.2km)	255	340	425
10000 (7km)	345	457	572
15000 (10.5km)	515	687	858
20000 (14km)	687	915	1144
*Based on 10000 steps = 7km walking. Adjust figures for your own data on how far you walk in 10000 steps.			

Speed of Results

The expected Speed of results can be worked out from using rough calorie calculations. The classic model of calories assumes there are 7700 calories in a KG of body fat (3500 cals/pound). Therefore, to lose 1 kg of body fat you need to create a deficit of 7700 calories over a specific time period. Using this data you can then gauge some actual realistic expectations on how long it takes to lose body fat. The following table shows the expected time scales for fat loss based on the calorie deficit and expected level of difficulty.

Calorie Deficit / Day	Expected Fat Loss / week*	Difficulty
100	0.1 kg	Easy**
250	0.22kg	Easy – Average
500	0.45 kg	Average
750	0.7 kg	Average – Hard
1000	0.95 kg	Hard
1500	1.40 kg	Very Hard
2000	1.8 kg	Nearly Impossible
3000	2.7 kg	Nearly Impossible
*Genuine fat loss amounts, the scales may give different readings		
**Fat loss is never easy per se but refers to the metabolic demand		

Do not live by these numbers, they are general estimates to be used as a guide. There are many factors that affect the process such as your varying energy needs and total food consumed. There is also the issue around how much a genuine loss in body fat shows itself on the weighing scales.

The same data applies to gaining body fat as well, you do not magically gain lots of body fat because you ate a chocolate bar. If you consistently over eat then the expected numbers would start applying to you. This data does not apply to short term eating periods. The expected time scales for results that account for behaviour change are discussed in the section 3.

Metabolic Adaption

One of the issues with treating the body as a pure calorie calculator is that we fundamentally assume it is constant. This is not the case in the real world, we have already discussed how your daily calorie needs can vary based on the temperatures of your environment, the menstrual cycle or stress levels amongst others factors as well as how much you move. This already makes it hard to say if you are definitely 100, 300 or 500 calories under your needs.

Another issue is called metabolic adaption, which is how your body adjusts its own calorie requirements. Your body has the ability to adjust its calorie needs up or down. This is important in conversations around calorie deficits and speed of results.

As you lose weight over a prolonged period of time the body will try to prevent losses by reducing your calorie needs. This can be done in various ways, e.g. lowering body temperature (this is why you can feel cold when dieting). This generally means as you lose body fat your numbers will probably have to change. You will need to gradually decrease calorie intake or increase movement. This will not be dramatic in that you need to drop your food intake by a third overnight but more subtle. You will also need to factor in that if you weigh less the same amount of movement or exercise uses less energy.

In the real world you can counter some of this by taking breaks from losing body fat, not using extreme calorie deficits and also getting fitter during the process. If you are fitter in three months then you will be inclined to move more which will offset the reduced energy needs.

When you finish your diet and begin eating at break-even thresholds again your metabolic rate will begin to rise as you are now eating adequate amounts of food.

Your metabolic rate may return back to previous levels but often it will be slightly lower than before. Some of this is metabolic adaption while some is due to you weighing less.

Metabolic adaption is often unavoidable. This is shown by how someone who has lost weight will need less calories than a person of the same size that has never had to lose weight. However, the differences are not usually huge in that perhaps you need just 100 or 200 calories a day less. They also do not apply to everybody which is due to genetics.

Metabolism as a Wave

So far we have been talking about losing fat all in terms of numbers without any reference to the real world difficulty of how hard it is to follow a plan or sustain a calorie deficit.

We have discussed already how it is sensible to view your body and your behaviours as slightly different and apart from YOU the person. I used the analogy of a horse to represent your body & behaviours with YOU being the rider.

When it comes to metabolism and fat loss I like to use a different metaphor. A more appropriate way to view your body during fat loss is that you are a surfer and your metabolism is the sea. Your goal is to ride to the waves to get to shore.

Why a wave? For starters, it shows that your metabolism is not fixed or constant but it is changing and unpredictable. As you enter a calorie deficit and begin under eating you engage the body defences against famine. Initially this is very subtle and barely noticeable. However, as you progress forwards and lose body fat it begins to build. This is accelerated if you greatly under eat compared to your calorie needs. As time passes your hunger increases, your motivation weakens and your energy levels become much more variable.

This is akin to the wave getting bigger and bigger. As days and weeks progress you may find the wave gets so big it crushes you and knocks you off the board. This could mean you binge for a few days, quit your exercise programme or maybe you get sick with a cold.

At this point you may become demotivated and question why you cannot stick to the plan, you feel down, guilty and angry. But does a surfer really feel guilty for a wave knocking them off the board? Why not blame the wave? This whole issue is compounded if you use the weighing scales to monitor progress as you will see a rapid increase in weight from stored carbohydrates, water and food within the digestive system after eating too much.

However, you have done nothing wrong! The only mistake you made was thinking you are in control of metabolism. Surfers fall off waves all the time, just gather yourself and jump back on the next wave when you are ready.

The body will give you signs about how it is reacting. This comes in the form of energy, motivation, hunger, how the body feels and how quickly body fat is changing. This will give you a clue about how the wave is building and if it is time to get off, take a break and wait for the next one.

Calories Intake & Reactions

When you know that you cannot just create a calorie deficit and lose fat without experiencing other reactions it gives a greater understanding of the biochemistry involved in changing your body. The following table gives a generalised schema about the expected reactions based on how much you have under eaten:

Deficit	Speed of Results	Difficulty	Sustainability*
10%	Slow	Easy**	Many Months
20%	Moderate	Moderate	~1 Month
30%	Moderate / Fast	Moderate/Hard	Few Weeks
40%	Fast	Hard	~1 Week
50%+	Very Fast	Very Hard	Days

*Time before taking a break at maintenance, varies on many factors
**Fat loss is never easy per se but refers to the metabolic demand

As you can see in the chart, as the size of the calorie deficit increases, the demands on you and your body does as well. For example, let's say you need 2000 calories a day based on your metabolism and the movement you are doing. Eating 1800 a day would represent a 10% deficit all things being equal. This would produce slow steady fat loss, it would not be a huge tax on the body and you wouldn't expect huge craving to occur or big energy dips etc.

If you adopted a 50% deficit and ate 1000 calories a day you would see rapid fat loss in that you could see yourself thinner every few days. However, you would also experience big swings in energy, strong food cravings and changes in mood. Your sleep may become disturbed and you would find it hard to stick to. You would need very high motivation to sustain it.

Neither approach is better, some people prefer a 10% undercut while others go harder then take a break through structured off days or weeks back at maintenance. We shall discuss these methods later on. What is important for you to understand is that the laws are fairly immutable.

Under eating brings with it consequences that have nothing to do with how motivated you are or what you would like to achieve. It works independently of you as it is routed in biology. How you handle these inevitable side effects of fat loss will determine results.

You will not truly know what your exact percentage undercut is because you cannot know your exact energy needs or how your body reacts to fat loss by changing your metabolism.

You may see someone losing fat eating a lot more food than you or likewise see someone eating so much less. Do not worry or get caught up in comparing yourself to them. You do not know how their metabolism functions compared to yours. You just need to find out and use the ideal amounts for you.

Calorie Thresholds

The last few segments hopefully have given insight into the fat loss process, the expected speed of change and how you may feel during it. It also would have given you a little understanding of the numbers involved in energy balance and the quirks of the body that can manipulate it.

At a practical level I find it helpful to use the concept of calorie thresholds. These are points at which you generally start to see certain reactions happen. The three main thresholds are show below –

Calories

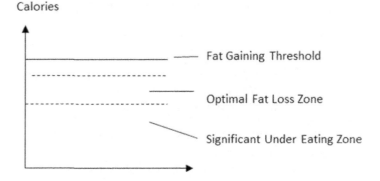

The fat gaining threshold is where you start to accumulate body fat. This is fairly easy to reach if eating 'junk' foods and still possible though harder to do when eating 'clean' food or a healthy diet.

Your aim is to find the optimal fat loss zone, which is when you are losing body fat yet have the energy to function in life. You are not suffering long periods of hunger or big energy crashes. The process is manageable and suits your mind set.

Even when you are within this optimal fat loss zone you will still need to take a break from the plan at some point. This is to avoid being crushed by the wave of metabolism that builds up as you lose more and more body fat. The larger your deficit the more often you will need to take a break. Whether your optimal zone is a larger or smaller deficit is mix of personal preference vs how your body reacts.

When you drift too low in calorie intake you will enter into the significant under eating zone. Here you will find that your energy starts to drop, your cravings increase and your willpower is lowered. In this region the plan is unsustainable. Eventually you will break the diet and often in spectacular fashion.

The above thresholds show the general calorie intake levels over a week assuming movement stays constant. For most people this is all you need to know for getting results

*****

While explaining fat loss we have talked about calorie intake and calorie numbers etc. Please understand you do <u>not</u> need to be counting calories every day to get results. The energy balance mechanism is working all the time whether you think about it or not. There are many ways to create a calorie deficit without weighing your foods. I merely use the term calories as it is the most scientific way to discuss and explain food intake amounts.

Where Does Body Fat Disappear From?

Another concept to understand is where body fat comes from once you have successfully created a calorie deficit. This is very important as most people are awful at seeing changes within their own body. This can cause you to quit because you have not seen results even though you have actually lost fat.

Your body stores excess fat either under the skin, within the muscles or around your organs. As mentioned before, where you store your fat is mostly genetic and it varies amongst the population. To answer the question of where do you lose fat from you need to go back to when you first started gaining it.

As you first began to gain body fat (this could have been a long time ago) your body put it into what you probably now describe as your worst areas. As fat continued to increase over time it would have spread it around the body a bit more while still putting a fair bit in your worst areas.

Continued fat gain after this point would see it go to the organs (this is called visceral fat) and yet more fat gain after this would see the whole body accumulate fat in all areas with significant amounts going to your worst bits and the organs.

The fat loss process happens mostly in reverse order. Your body is usually very keen to get rid of fat off the organs so early fat loss will often look to take it from this area. However, fat is never taken from just one place. It always comes from a mixture of different areas.

While organ fat loss is good for your health you cannot see your liver so it does not change your appearance. As far as other areas of initial fat loss you can almost guarantee that it comes from areas you do not care about that much. Your fat may come from already quite lean areas, for example, you lose it off your feet or your hands but not your worst areas.

In general, you probably underestimate how much body fat you have because much of it is subtly hidden as your whole body gets bigger. When you look at yourself for example, you may look at how much your stomach is sticking out in front of your legs. However, you do not notice the fact your legs have got bigger themselves so you actually have more fat than you thought.

Overtime, your body will take body fat from every area and all your worst bits. The key is patience and persistence. If you are say 8% from your body fat goal, the first 3% of fat loss may not come from any of your worst bits. Then the next 3% may take a little from your worst bits but also other areas. Finally, the last 2% may be from your very worst spots.

Noticing Body Fat Losses

The inability to notice body fat losses is a problem. To get around this issue you must look at the whole body including areas which are already lean so you can spot changes.

Fat loss will show itself with subtle changes. This could be seeing more veins in your arms or on the body, noticing lines of shadow or striations in the muscles appearing. You may feel the bones in your feet or hands become more prominent. Your rings may become looser, face appears thinner etc. These are all subtle signs that you are losing body fat. If you continue the process you will eventually see losses from your worst bits. Avoid looking only at your worst areas.

Health Issues & Blocking Factors

One area around the fat loss mechanism to consider is the effect of health issues and blocking factors on losing body fat.

Health issues include conditions such PCOS, diabetes, low thyroid, hormonal imbalances (e.g. menopause), ME, Chronic fatigue and a host of other possible issues.

Blocking factors refer to things that affect health such as metabolic syndrome, adrenal fatigue, Leptin sensitivity, food allergies or the medications you are taking and their side effects.

The influences of health traits and blocking factors on the fat loss process are a source of great debate. On the one side they are given as a reason why someone cannot lose body fat. This is backed up by the difficulty experienced by the individuals and the research studies showing correlations between health problems, medication use and weight issues.

The counter arguments to this come from those pointing out you cannot change the underlying physical laws of energy and thermodynamics which means anyone can lose weight. There are also examples of individuals who get results despite having these same health issues and blocks.

As so often is the case both sides have a point. You cannot change thermodynamics but you can have health issues and blocking factors cause havoc with your fat loss attempts. The key here is where they are acting within the fat loss process. They do not alter the underlying rules of energy balance but they do influence the factors within the energy balance equation that we have discussed already. Any health condition or blocking factor could affect energy balance by –

Reducing Your Metabolic Rate – One way many issues act upon your body is by decreasing your metabolic strength, for example the thyroid gland can influence 10% of your base calorie expenditure. So a thyroid issue may reduce your metabolic rate by 3% for example. Many medications and health conditions will have this effect upon your metabolism. The lower your calorie needs the less food you need per day so the easier it becomes to gain weight and more difficult it is to lose body fat.

Decreasing Your Desire to Move –Another pathway by which these issues can interfere with the process is by decreasing your overall energy levels or increasing pain within the body. This makes it less likely you will want to move. If this is prolonged then your fitness levels will drop greatly and you will move even less. This is compounded by a general society that is moving less and becoming more overweight.

Increasing Desire to Eat – A further possible route is through changes in food cravings, increased hunger and alterations in the fullness mechanism when you are eating. Various medications can increase hunger and any issues that increases pain, worry or makes you feel down is likely to increase comfort eating. The more you want to eat the harder it is to maintain your weight or lose fat.

Interrupting Your Behaviour / Thought Patterns – The final possible mechanism is through changes in your behaviour patterns and thinking. For example, if you are in pain or depressed then it is unlikely you will have much energy or desire to be thinking about changing your body shape. This will therefore influence your results.

*****

One or all of these influences can affect your ability to lose body fat. It could be your PCOS means you feel pain and low energy which makes you move less which is on top of your metabolic rate being slower than it used to be. This makes it tougher for you to get in shape.

Perhaps the new medications you are taking have increased hunger and you have started to comfort eat more because of your worries about your health issues.

Maybe the unexplained joint pain you are suffering has meant you can no longer go for a run and as a result you are out of your health routine. Instead of jogging and feeling good you end up feeling down while watching TV and eating.

These influences make it so much harder for some people to get in shape than others. Even though it may be difficult It is important to understand that it is not biochemically impossible. We know this is true because you can find examples of people with the same issues who have lost body fat and not everyone on medications associated with weight gain actually put on body fat. The energy balance equation and process still holds true. This is good to know because it means it is possible to achieve your goals.

Fat Loss Myths & Inaccuracies

The final thing to look at around fat loss is to clarify some of the lies and inaccuracies that you may have commonly heard being discussed.

The Placebo Effect & Bad Science

One of the reasons that weight loss has become so mystical these days is due to both the placebo effect, which is the tendency for the body to react to an action simply because the person believes it will have a benefit and the application of bad scientific practices.

This is important as both of these behaviours result in people incorrectly attributing certain actions as a cause of fat loss when really it was the old standard basics of manipulating the energy balance equation.

My one friend swears she can only lose weight by having lemon juice in the morning. Whenever she does this she also cuts out obvious junk food from her diet and makes sure she hits 15000 steps a day. She always loses body fat this way and then credits the lemon juice for helping her metabolism.

This is both bad science and the placebo effect in action. In the real world lemon juice does not speed up metabolism and I could easily try to convince her she was wrong. I could bombard her with facts to prove that I am right. However, If I really wanted to help her lose weight... It would be easier to just buy her some lemons.

The fat loss game is littered with these sorts of stories, beliefs and superstitions. If a placebo behaviour is within a good sound plan of action there is nothing wrong with them.

Where they becomes a problem is when a placebo story is added to other placebo stories and before long you have lost sight of all the basics that actually gets results. The end result could be some lunatic plan where you need to drink a cup green tea followed by a two minute headstand and then do backward walking for five minutes to lose weight. Solid plans of action always come back to energy balance and the behaviours behind creating an ongoing calorie deficit.

Different Methodologies & Their Effectiveness

There are so many methods and approaches to losing body fat. Whatever the methodology, it will create results through doing one of the following –

Decreasing Food Intake – Most plans to lose weight simply cut down food intake, usually by replacing higher calorie dense foods with lower ones like vegetables and lean protein. This makes it much harder to overeat.

Decreasing Your Desire to Eat – The need to eat can be reduced by changing the food within your diet, increasing motivation, changing your behaviours around eating or reducing stress. This is why yoga and meditation, despite burning so few calories in a session can be great for fat loss as you eat less when you are more relaxed.

Increasing Movement – Most exercise plans are based on getting you to move and burn calories. As discussed, a plan does not have to use formal exercise as any increase in activity or movement will use energy and aid in fat loss.

Increasing Your Desire to Move – The more appealing any form of movement appears the greater the likelihood of you doing it. Many fitness approaches use this type of approach including dance, Zumba and different novelty workouts.

Increasing Metabolism – Some plans and strategies actively work on trying to increase metabolism. This will of course contribute to the energy balance equation.

Placebo Effect on Actions – As mentioned, the placebo effect of believing something works makes people do more of the right behaviours that they know they should be doing and less of the bad ones they should avoid.

All effective fat loss plans work by manipulating your energy balance over a prolonged period of time. The key is how can you sustain such a plan? You will learn more about this in the next section.

Fat Loss Myths

The following methods are things that you do <u>not have to do</u> to lose weight. You may choose to do some of these if it appeals but it is not necessary. These myths often stem from people trying to sell you a product using that particular methodology or because they like it themselves. Some of the biggest myths include;

No Carbs – You can lose fat with carbohydrates. Everyone lost weight eating carbs back in the 1980s when low fat diets were the trend. Despite the perception many bodybuilders compete while eating carbs, Carbs are fine!

Keto – You do not need to be in a keto state to lose fat, do you really think if you ate only 4 bananas a day (500 calories) you wouldn't lose weight because you are not in keto?

Not Eating at Night – You can eat anytime of the day, every year millions of Muslims lose weight during Ramadan when they only eat at night time. If the food amount stays the same it does not matter what time you eat it.

Cut Out Your Favourite Foods – You can eat your favourite foods and still lose weight. The key is ensuring you do not go crazy on them so the energy balance equation still holds true.

Eat Only Salad – There is more to life than salad, in fact, most people who eat only salad while trying to lose fat end up eating so little food they get crushed by the wave of their metabolism and end up binge eating.

Eat Vegetables & Low Calorie Foods – You do not necessarily have to eat low calorie foods or vegetables. It is about getting the energy balance right which can still be done with higher calorie foods as long as you are aware of overall intake.

Intermittent Fasting – There is no magic in not eating during a certain part of the day. You can lose fat eating every three hours or avoiding food for sixteen hours. It is a personal choice and not something you have to do.

Carb Cycling – You can lose fat with carbs in the diet, without them in your diet (keto) or by cycling them in and out. You do not need to do it though.

Nutrient Timing – You can eat anytime you like as long as you have a negative energy balance to lose body fat.

Eat Clean – No Junk Food – You do not have to eat clean foods, cut out wheat or stop junk food to lose fat. You just need to ensure that the higher calorie foods that come with these foods do not disrupt your calorie deficit.

No Sugar – You can lose fat with sugar in the diet just like you can lose fat with carbohydrates. All carbs turn into sugar the moment you digest it anyhow. People were losing fat way before everyone became scared of sugar.

Fat Burners – You do not need to take a fat burner, they barely make a dent on your metabolic rate and even if they do, they usually increase your hunger by the same amount. This means you are in the same situation as before. The more serious fat burners that some bodybuilders use are the ones that kill people. These have serious consequences! You do <u>not</u> need fat burners to lose fat.

Believe in Results – You do not need to believe in results or success. You just need to do the actions that create change.

Body Type Based Nutrition – You do not have to follow a specific nutrition plan because of your body type. Regardless of what any test may say you can work around it and lose body fat if you get the energy balance right. For example, you take a test that says you need to eat lots of animal protein yet you are vegan…. Relax! You can still lose body fat without eating meat. The more a plan is tailored to your body the easier it is. However, I would suggest listening to how your body reacts for this feedback over some random report.

Cortisol – Your Cortisol issues are not preventing you from losing body fat. I used to test people's adrenal function. It was always those with lowest Cortisol levels who had the most body fat and not the other way round. Cortisol is slow to change its basic pattern and cannot explain why you lose fat one week and not the next, or vice versa.

Hormones – Your hormones are not preventing you losing fat. They can influence you in others areas such as desire to eat or strength of metabolism as discussed before. However, if you set the energy balance to create a deficit you will lose fat.

Go Hard With Hiit – People were losing body fat way before Hiit was even invented. You do not have to do it!

Fat Loss Cardio Zone – You can lose fat doing Hiit, which is way above the fat loss burning zone, or by walking slowly which is below it. You do not need the fat loss cardio zone.

Fasted Cardio – It does not matter what time you eat or exercise, it is the balance of energy that determines results.

EPOC – You do not need to worry about increasing EPOC, the extra energy burnt after exercise. You can lose fat by walking and modifying food if you wanted to which has no EPOC.

Micronutrients – You can lose fat without adequate vitamin or mineral intake. This is what happens in a famine. Optimising health and losing body fat is not the same thing. Ideally you would meet all your nutrient needs of course.

Set Points – The various set point theories suggest as your body fat gets to a certain low level it increases hunger and decreases metabolism making it harder or impossible to lose more body fat.

Personally I believe the set point theory can be almost entirely explained as a psychological process over one of physiology within the body. It is an interesting debate though when discussing bodybuilders nearing shows when they have super low levels of body fat. For almost everyone this issue is irrelevant as your goal will be above any set point that may exist. The argument for set points at higher more normal body fat ranges is unconvincing. You are not trapped by your physiology. You can lose body fat.

Eat less and less – You do not need to keep trying to reduce your food intake further and further. You just need to set the food intake level against your movement so you can lose fat. This should be done in a sustainable way which may mean regular fat loss breaks.

Move More and More – You do not need to keep increasing how much you move. You are trying to create a calorie deficit you can sustain. So you need to move the appropriate amount to create the deficit based on your food intake.

Eat Nothing to Maintain Your Results – You do not need to eat tiny amounts of food to maintain your goal body fat. This is a fallacy, assuming you are breaking even now before you start the process then all of the bad behaviours you are currently doing can also be done to maintain your body fat levels when you reach your goal.

While your metabolic rate may drop if you lose a lot of weight it is usually fairly small differences, e.g. 100 or 200 calories less / day. Some of this is because you weigh less so you use less energy during movement as you are lighter. It is important you understand the fat loss protocol you use is not the maintenance plan. You can eat more and move less to break even. Sustaining your results is significantly easier than you imagine. You do not need to be a saint.

*****

As we leave the mechanics of fat loss behind, I must remind you again that results are not just about fat loss knowledge. They are about how you manage your own emotions, behaviours and actions to be able to change your body. Looking at body shape and transformation as just calories in vs out is too simplistic and needs to be accompanied by the changes behind the scenes.

I keep mentioning this because you will probably find yourself falling back into this simplistic model of thinking that it is just a physical or mechanical issue. It is natural for us to do that.

The Grand Unified Theory of Weight Loss

How Do You Gain Muscle

Developing muscle is central to many people's goals, this could be as part of the toning up process or as the main focus of your entire programme if you are looking to add significant amounts of muscle. It is vital to understand the mechanics of muscle growth so you can optimise your results.

On the following pages I will detail how you can develop your muscle all the way up to that of a bodybuilder or anywhere in between. As mentioned with fat loss, remember that techniques and knowledge are only part of the solution to your goals. It is the prolonged application of the behaviours that gets results which is based on your thinking patterns.

This is especially true in this area as it can take many years to achieve your end goal if you want add a lot of muscle. Note - If you do not want to gain muscle then skip this section.

The Stimulus to Create New Muscle –

The very first stage of muscle growth is generating a stimulus for the body to create new muscle tissue. To do this you must make the muscles move against a slightly harder than usual resistance. While this could simply come from doing the gardening, if you want to be adding noticeable amounts of muscle it needs to be from a resistance training routine in some form.   Resistance training is not just lifting weights in the gym. It can be using your own body weight at home or more gymnastic forms such as pole dancing or bar calisthenics.

What defines resistance training is how you do the exercise. The movement needs to create fatigue or stress within the muscles roughly between 1- 20 repetitions (5-60 seconds duration) followed by a rest long enough to allow some partial recovery.

It is important to reach the right intensity, just having a dumbbell does not mean you are doing resistance training. You will struggle to build any muscle if doing weight training with a weight that is so light you could lift it easily for 50+ reps. On the flipside, aerobic exercise can build muscle if you are doing short intense bursts, this is seen with cyclists who grow big legs muscles from hill climbs and flat sprints which represent resistance training type activities.

Maintaining the Stimulus to Grow Muscle

It is easy to create a stimulus for muscle growth, especially for people new to exercise. What is more difficult is maintaining it as you progress and add more muscle.

Let's walk through how it may look for a typical person. The first day you do any exercise you could probably create a stimulus for muscle growth by doing just one set of 10 repetitions, e.g. 10 push ups or 10 squats. Do an exercise for all of the major muscle groups and you have done a nice workout. It may only take you 10 minutes to do.

This short workout sent a stimulus to grow muscle which lasts for a couple of days. At this point you do another exercise session by doing the same workout again. By keeping this pattern going you soon find that you feel stronger (this is initially through the brain learning to recruit your muscles better) and thus you increase the weights used to match this extra strength. This process is then repeated and you will very slowly begin growing muscle.

After a period of time the body will become used to this 10 reps, 1 set / major muscle group workout. You will still work up a sweat but you will no longer be increasing strength or size. At this point you have to change something to force the body to send out a signal to create new muscle. If you did not want to dedicate more than 10 minutes you could simply change the number of reps you are doing, perhaps do half the number of reps and make all the weights heavier so you reach fatigue after 5 reps and not 10. This would create a new challenge and once more your body would send the signal to create new muscle tissue.

At some point after this your body will become accustomed to the stimulus and once more you will need to change something. Maybe you change the exercises that you use for each body part, perhaps you alter the speed and tempo of the lift. This will again restart the muscle building process. You can continue adjusting the programme and finding ways to keep the body sending out a signal for new muscle tissue.

However, eventually you will get to the stage where you have done all that you can on your current volume of workout (10 minutes). You would now have to go from doing 1 set to 2 sets / muscle group. You could then employ all the methods you used previously to continue to make muscle gains on your now 20 minute routine.

Over time this routine would also no longer produce a stimulus to grow and you would have to increase the routine from 2 sets to 3 sets / major muscle. This cycle repeats itself over and over so eventually you would need to go up to 4, then 5 sets. The end point of this process is that you either achieve your muscle goals so you can remain at that particular volume or you need to find a way to add yet more sets.

The problem of such an increasingly long programme is either you cannot dedicate the time per session to do the higher volume or you reach the edge of how much quality lifting you can do before fatigue sets in and ruins the workout.

Split Routines

A split routine refers to how many days it takes to work all the major muscles on the body. A 1 day split means you do all your body parts on one day, e.g. legs, arms, chest etc. Alternatively, a 3 day split means you work every muscle part over three days, e.g. Day 1 - pushing muscles like chest, shoulders and triceps. Day 2 - pulling muscles of the back and biceps. Day 3 – Legs and abdominal work.

As the sets per muscle group increase you will eventually need to use a split routine in some form. This allows you to put in quality work to stimulate more muscle growth. The key to using split routine is consistency. You would be training at least 3 times a week to use a split of some sort but ideally 4-5+ times. You will struggle to get results using a split routine if you often miss training sessions. They need consistency.

How Long Do the Muscle Stimulus Cycles Last?

This is a difficult question to answer but the general rule of thumb is 3 to 4 weeks. However, it depends on how much you have changed the programme. There are significant individual differences with some people being much more responsive than others.

You should look at your results, e.g. are you still getting stronger, to give you a clue about how you are progressing. Your interest, enthusiasm and motivation to your programme should also be considered. As muscle growth is so slow it can be hard to use the mirror as your only guide.

You should not rush through the muscle stimulus cycles. The best way to progress is to make use of your early training status and extracting the muscle growth from lower volume amounts while you can. If you dive straight in at 5 sets per muscle group you will miss out on numerous easier and shorter opportunities to grow muscle.

The 5 sets per muscle programme will not magically add new amounts of muscle tissue at twice the speed because you jumped the earlier steps. It does not accelerate the timeframe of results. This is why so many people fail to build muscle. They are not patient and try to jump ahead and take short cuts. Muscle building is about patience, persistence and consistency.

Advanced Lifting Techniques

The following elements are important for advanced lifters;

Frequency - When it comes to adding significant muscle size almost everyone is training 4-6 times a week in a gym. For modest muscle building goals you could probably achieve it on 1 -3 resistance sessions per week. However, to enter the realms of adding serious muscle you will eventually need to be up in this higher frequency range.

Do not be put off by this thought, the build-up from lifting nothing or inconsistently to needing 4-6 times a week would probably take 1–3 years if not longer.

Effort – One of the keys to muscle building success is training hard with high levels of effort. This is often incorrectly referred to as intensity*, or high intensity effort.

Training with a lot of effort, focus and determination can greatly extend the time period you can build muscle on lower volumes and smaller split routines.

For experienced lifters, effort is an essential element to create a stimulus for building new muscle tissue. This is why bodybuilding is such a difficult sport. Each set needs to bring with it effort and an inevitable pain. This refers to a good pain of burning / fatigue within the muscles.

It is very hard to keep yourself mentally focused set on set, session on session and not quit when the pain kicks in. This comes back to the many factors we will discuss later on around motivation, focus and how to raise your standards.

(*Intensity officially refers to the weight lifted compared to your maximum possible lift. This means 3 sets of 2 reps with the heaviest weight you can lift with 5 minutes rest is a much higher intensity lift than 3 sets of 12 reps with 1 minute rest. However, the pain and discomfort in the sets of 12 reps will be much greater than 2 reps. This has led to confusion between efforts in lifting (trying hard/pain experienced) and high intensity workloads (heaviest you can lift for lower reps). High effort with medium intensity ranges (5-15 reps) develops muscle maximally and is more painful than true high intensity.

Muscle Activation Techniques – Muscle development in bodybuilding circles has a huge emphasis on recruiting the whole muscle length. As your muscle size increases your future development will become hindered by the smallest part of the muscle.

Just doing an exercise is unlikely to activate and develop the whole muscle, rather it will focus specifically on one part of the muscle area, e.g. the bench press does your lower outside chest. As that part grows over time, further chest development may become limited because of the lack of development in your upper and lower inside chest size. At this point you need to change the focus of your chest work to bring up these laggings areas within the muscle.

The problem you have is that the strong part of your chest is ready and super excited to do any lifting it can. This means you will often find that whatever exercise you choose you cannot develop the weaker areas because of this dominance.

The way around this is selecting the right exercise variations that make it easier for the body to pick the lagging area. In combination you would use mind muscle recruitment to think it into activating more. Any bodybuilders with good muscle mass will have a very well developed sense of mind muscle connection.

Even with the right exercises and mental focus you may well find that you struggle to activate the muscles correctly, especially early or late within a lifting motion where the muscle is longest or shortest.

Muscle Integrity Development – One of the reasons you are unable to activate specific muscles or parts of a muscle is due to the quality of the muscle tissue itself.

Muscle integrity refers to how smooth and well aligned the muscle tissue is, this include knots and lumps within it as well as scar tissue from previous injuries. When you have areas of lower integrity tissue it is hard for blood to get into them and therefore it is difficult to activate the area.

Using massage techniques is important when trying to improve activation. A sports massage therapist is by far the most effective method you could use but other viable options include self-massage, massage guns, lacrosse balls, foam rollers or stretching.

After improving the muscle tissue you will find you are better able to activate the sleeping parts of muscles and improve your mind muscle connection. This can really help with the more stubborn muscles that refuse to grow.

Often the inability to recruit certain muscles is due to the joint being in the wrong postural position while lifting. Very subtle changes in joint angle will increase or decrease the activation of certain muscles. These distorted postures are often caused by areas with poor integrity pulling the joint out of alignment and/or through overactive muscles. The use of massages can realign good joint angle through releasing spasms and down regulating overactive muscles. This will also aid in waking up sleeping muscles to support the joint.

A related feature to muscle integrity is fascia health. The fascia is a see through sheath that goes around the muscle. Different fascia sheaths are connected to each other so they have a role to play in correcting joint alignment.

In muscle building terms some people have much tighter fascia which squeezes the muscle and make them look smaller than they area. Fascia based stretching or massage can create changes in body shape and apparent size.

Body Part Emphasis – As you develop more muscle over time you will always find certain body parts lag behind. Your split routine needs to encompass particular focus for a lagging body part as well as exercises to target the weak muscle areas

By emphasising a muscle while still developing other areas you can bring out parts of your body that were lagging. This can take a few months to half a year or more to resolve a very difficult area. You will still develop the whole body where you can but the focus is on bringing up the smaller areas.

This stems from bodybuilding shows where you are judged on the relative proportion of muscle sizes. While most people do not want to be a bodybuilder understanding lagging body parts can really accelerate the transformation process as a big element of appearance is where you gain the muscle and not just how much muscle is added.

Progressive Overload for Advanced Lifters

The key to muscle growth is creating a stimulus to grow and then repeating it again and again overtime. When you do this you will make ongoing progress and continued muscle gains.

When you reach the maximum threshold of training where you are in the gym 5-6 days a week you cannot just keep adding in more sessions or dedicating more time.

At this point it is a real skill to keep your body progressing and sending out signals to grow more muscle tissue. One way to do this is to ensure you keep your lifting effort high. This is very hard to do session in session out which is why most people struggle to grow large amounts of muscle. The other way is to make clever use of exercise variation over time with different split routines, targeted exercise techniques and alterations in the rest, rep and lifting tempo.

The advice at this stage is what fills the heads of top bodybuilding coaches and the serious lifters. This applies only to a small percentage of athletes. Most people can achieve their goals with what has been outlined already. Achieving higher level performance require specific programs tailored to you. There is no general magic formula to copy as you need to find what programme, schema and food protocols maximise your results. This varies greatly between individuals.

Speed of Muscle Gain

The reason so many struggle with gaining muscle is the demoralising speed of progress. Even when you do everything right it takes time to see results. Genuine muscle gains may average around 1-2Kg per year, especially as you advance and gain more muscle. While individual differences exist and the use of steroids will accelerate the process it is always slow.

Muscle gains rely on faith that the training will produce the results. You will also need an enjoyment of the process and doing the exercise sessions. Without these it is unlikely you will stick to it long enough to see results.

Depending on your goals, it could take five years to get to your end goal if you did everything right. This is in contrast to fat loss, where at 1% fat loss per week you could have everyone commenting on how you look slimmer within a month and leave everyone shocked with your transformation after three months. Fat loss is much faster than muscle gain.

Where Do You Gain Muscle?

In general you will gain muscle in the places where you have been working the muscles. This does not mean you have to do an exercise for each muscle on the body as exercises can activate many muscles at the same time. However, as you get bigger you will need to target more specific parts of muscles for continued growth.

The general rule of thumb is that you should feel a burn in the muscle area you want to grow. The body part should become pumped during the session and it is common to feel stiffness in the area (especially when first targeting it). It is <u>not</u> necessary to feel stiff the next day to build muscle.

Muscle Gain & Appearance

There are a few elements to understand in regards to how muscle influences how you look. These include;

Non Linear Relationship of Muscle to Appearance – The visual changes you see via muscle gain are non-linear. Initial gains in muscle do not make a huge difference in appearance. However when you already have a lot of muscle a moderate gain of 1 or 2kg can really change how you look.

A good way to picture this is that you start off as an empty flat balloon. Your muscle represents the air inside and your appearance is the actual size of the balloon. As you begin to put some air into it, you initially do not see much change in overall size. In fact, it barely seems like anything is changing. As a bit more air goes in, eventually a certain part of the balloon expands but it is not that impressive to someone who wants a balloon for their birthday party.

A little more air goes in and it is now fully formed in shape but it is small and soft. However, all future air put into it will now create noticeable increases in the size of the balloon. The last few inputs of air really increase the size of the balloon. Muscle gain follows this pattern, slow to start with faster visual gains towards the end.

Muscles in Specific Places Make a Huge Difference – Muscle gain for most people is not just about adding muscle for no reason. It is usually done to look more muscular or to be stronger or both. When it comes to looking muscular there is a skill and an art to knowing where to grow muscle tissue.

We do not evaluate people just on muscle mass or weight, we instead look at the relative proportions of certain muscles versus other muscles. For example, your arms are more noticeable than your hamstrings.

It gets more subtle than that though. If you were to gain 0.5kg of muscle on your chest, you would appear more muscular to the naked eye if you added that muscle to the upper chest rather than the lower chest. This is because most people are already lower chest dominant and adding it higher up will form a line down the middle of the body which gets interpreted as you being bigger. This is the basis of physique competitions, relative sizes of different parts of the muscle and muscle groups across the body.

If you gained 3 kg of muscle just on your thighs (e.g. from cycling) the change in your appearance would be much less than if you gained 3kg spread out across your chest, shoulders and arms.

This sort of specific body part development really becomes important once you have gained a nice amount of muscle already. Early stages where you are still getting the body to take shape it is not so important.

However, using a solid foundation from day 1 will create more even muscle development and you will accelerate results. All of this specificity and focus is straight out of bodybuilding. It is not just about lifting, grunting or taking steroids. It is a very subtle but skilful sport.

Size - Body Fat vs Muscle Mass – One problem you get when chasing size and getting bigger is the confusion between what is muscle and what is body fat. How big you are is affected by both. As you gain body fat it goes all over the body, you can store body fat in the muscle tissues themselves as well as under the skin around the muscle.

If you have a good muscle base then the extra fat will make you look bigger and more muscular. However, your size is deceptive because how do you know how much is fat vs muscle? The only real way to know is to lose all your body fat and see what muscle you have left.

Most people have overestimated how much muscle they have compared to how much of it is body fat. This also shows itself when looking to add muscle. If you are making really quick progress so that you feel you are getting bigger week on week then you can almost guarantee you are just getting fatter. Genuine muscle gains are too slow to create such noticeable quick improvements.

Looking Ripped / Shredded – This refers to how much body fat you have vs your muscle mass. The '6 pack' is the symbolic muscle group of this term. Being ripped generally means you have low body fat which is showing off your muscles. The more muscle you have the higher your body fat can be for you to still be ripped. For example, if your abs muscles are small you six pack may only show at 8% body fat, if you have big abdominal muscles then maybe this same ripped look could happen at 14%.

As you lose body fat you will become smaller in actual size (circumferences of body parts) however you will look more muscular in photos or to the naked eye. This is because we judge muscularity by looking at the lines of shadow between muscles, their shape and other factors such as vascularity (how many veins you can see). All of these increase when you lose body fat.

How You Look Clothed Vs Naked - The desire to be big verses ripped is an ongoing consideration for most people who lift. This really shows itself when considering your optimal look for whether you are in or out of clothes.

Achieving a muscular look when dressed will be about filling the clothes out and overall size. In general the more body fat you have the bigger you will be which will make you look more muscular. If you have super low body fat you will be shredded but no one will know when you are covered up. Being super lean here can make you look thin in the face and the clothes can make you seems less muscular than you are.

When not wearing clothes, e.g. on a beach, achieving a muscular look will be about that shredded appearance. You would want a low body fat that would show off your muscles. It would make you appear bigger than your body actually is due to the lines of shadow and striations. If you had a lot of body fat, even though you may be muscly, with your top off you will look more overweight than muscular compared to the ripped person who has their abs showing.

There is no solution to these two ends of appearance. You will always be bigger in clothes with more body fat and always look more muscular when leaner when your body is on show. You should decide what is an acceptable range or an ideal mid-point. This will change over time as you gain muscle. If you are reliable and consistent with your ability to lose body fat then you could choose to have two different levels during the year, one for summer and one for winter. For most people though it is risky business to purposefully add body fat as they often never take it back off again.

Full vs Flat – A final element to consider with muscle and appearance is how optimised you look on any one day. The best you can look is if you have full carbohydrates stores, maximum hydration, your fascia and muscles are of high integrity (e.g. you just had a massage) and you have just done a total body workout to pump the muscles full of blood. In addition, you have not eaten for a few hours so the stomach is flat, you have a tan (if you are a lighter skin tone) and are looking at yourself under vertical lighting with a good pose. This is you looking your very best for that day. This is aided if you are on your own or next to people in 'worse' shape than yourself (they have less muscle or more body fat).

The other end to this scale and the worst you could look is when you have depleted your carb stores (after prolonged dieting) and you are dehydrated with tight muscles and fascia. In addition, you have not done any resistance training for a few days, you are untanned (if a lighter skin tone) and have just eaten a big meal to bloat your stomach. Finally you are in bright flat lighting and are not striking any sort of pose. This is you at your very worst for that day. This is compounded if you are next to people who are in much better shape than you (they have more muscle or less body fat).

These concepts are used all the time for photo shoots and bodybuilding shows. There is such a big difference between your best and worst look when you add in all of these factors. Social media makes use of the two conditions to exaggerate before and after body transformations. Most people's personal accounts are photos taken using most of the best photo scenarios. So which version of you is the true one?

The answer is neither, one of them is an over exaggeration and the other you are selling yourself short. While the truth may lie in the middle in day to day life you are more likely to believe the one that is most aligned to your beliefs or mood.

If you are in a good mood, or believe you are in good shape you are more likely to believe the "good" version of yourself. If you are in a bad mood or believe you have a bad body you will identify with the "bad" version.

This best vs worst image of you is wider problem around body image itself as it can really interfere with sensible self-evaluations. Many people get stuck on their worst version and exaggerate this to be even worse than it is in reality.

Consistency in evaluation is probably the key here so you can dissociate from having your evaluations controlled by your mood. This is best done alongside having a body positive approach of your current threshold of results.

Despite these issues there is a genuine difference between your "full" and "flat" versions in regards to how much muscle you appear to have. So it is important to understand this concept.

Protein and Calorie Intake

With the stimulus created to grow muscle from consistent resistance training and the progressive development of your plan you will now need to provide adequate protein and calorie intake for muscle growth.

The need to consume extra calories has been fairly exaggerated in general. One Kg of pure muscle contains less than 1000 calories, so if you took 2 months to gain a KG that would be just 15-20 calories per day extra[24]. This does not include the energy cost of making that muscle though. However, the point is that the energy needs for muscle gains are not huge. This makes sense really if you consider pregnant mothers need only 200 calories[25] extra per day during the last three months of pregnancy.

One factor to consider with calorie intake is how the body changes its metabolism when you eat more. As discussed previously your body can alter its metabolic rate. For example, if you need 2000 calories a day and thus eat 2030 calories to just give it those extra calories needed for muscle growth they could easily get used up by the body increasing your metabolism. So maybe you need to eat 200 calories more per day to ensure the body gets the extra 30 calories needed for muscle growth.

If you increase your calorie intake too much e.g. extra 1000-2000 calories / day, you will gain fat fairly quickly. You will know this because you will think you are growing muscle very quickly, which is not true. The advice to make huge increases in your food intake comes from bodybuilding where they use bulking and cutting cycles. The large calorie numbers they talk about are because they are huge people to start with and they are often taking industrial sized quantities of steroids which send the metabolic rate through the roof.

Protein wise, you will want to meet your needs but the more calories you eat the less protein you need for growth in general. This means most people think they need way more protein than they actually do. The high protein intakes are also pushed by some good marketing departments of the protein supplement companies. That being said, the average person's diet this day and age is deficient in protein so increasing your protein intake to even the lower suggested levels may seem a huge change in your routine.

Muscle can still be grown while losing fat when in a calorie deficit but under these circumstances protein intake becomes more important.

The general guide for protein intake would be at least 1g/Kg up to 2g/kg in a calorie surplus and 1.5g/kg to 2.5g/kg during a fat loss period[26]. For example, if you weigh 80kg you would want to eat between 120g or 200g per day of protein during a fat loss period. The science seems to suggest the upper limits listed above are perhaps a little high yet most people in bodybuilding circles would say they are too low. The answer lies in tailoring it to your own needs.

One point to note is that your body can use protein for your daily energy needs. It would be expected that people with much higher protein intakes than the ranges above are using more protein for fuel than the average person.

Bulking & Cutting Cycles

As most muscle gaining advice has come straight from professional bodybuilding the mantra of bulking and cutting still exists today.

A bulking period is where you purposely eat more food than you need to maximise muscle growth while accepting you will gain fat during the process. A cutting period is when you reduce food intake to lose the gained body fat from the bulk while maintaining muscle. Typically at the end of the cutting phase the physique competitor would enter a show.

While this method works for professional bodybuilders, for the average person it is a disaster. Even bodybuilders are using these cycles less than in previous times. The reason it does not work well is that you are probably not that good at losing body fat. This means you are taking a big risk to purposefully put on body fat which you may not be able to lose. The purported extra gains from the bulking cycle are also not that significant when you factor in the subsequent cutting period to get back to your ideal body fat range.

It is far more sensible to have more patience, eat a little more when trying to gain muscle but not to any great extent where body fat is going up quickly. Then periodically insert a fat loss period to ensure you do not creep too high in body fat.

Hormonal Environment

Assuming you are training and eating correctly as described the biggest determining factor on how much muscle you will gain is your hormonal environment.

There are big variations in hormones between individuals and most of this based on your genetics. There is not that much you can do about someone having better muscle potential than you but you can optimise your own levels. Regardless of your hormone profile everyone can gain significant amounts of muscle with time and patience. However, some can do it faster and to a greater extent.

The best way to help your own hormonal environment in the short term is to ensure you get adequate sleep each night (go to bed around 10pm and get 8 hours sleep) and remove any sensitive foods or toxic chemicals from your environment. Other factors that can help would be looking at breathing patterns & reducing stress.

A more medium to long term way to increase the hormonal environment is to do resistance training using some of the bigger whole body lifts such as deadlifts or squats. Over time you will become more responsive to hormones or increase your overall levels.

Any conversation about muscle and hormones of course brings up the topic of steroids. In general, most people use steroids too soon in their lifting timeline and then take too much of them to begin with. When added to the poor application of the basic mechanics of muscle gain many people get pretty average to poor results considering the risks they are taking. The vast majority of people can achieve their goals without ever using any performance enhancing drugs.

In general steroids get too much credit for results as you forget the effort, consistency, focus and dedication in training and nutrition that must come alongside them. For example, studies have shown that when given a placebo steroid, athletes increased their results greatly[27] despite not being on anything. This shows the influence of getting the basics inputs in place as previously discussed. This is shown also by how many people who are taking steroids get awful results and see few changes. You would never even suspect many steroid users were on them by looking at them.

That being said, if you have everything else in place, you have put in the time, the years and the effort to allow the body to grow from natural training progressions then steroids can take you to a level beyond natural limits and at much faster speeds. However, steroids bring many health risks that need to be considered.

Consistency & Patience

As you can see from all of the discussions so far on gaining muscle it is a very slow process. It is easy for you to quit before seeing results even though you are actually making good progress. It is important to be patient and continue training hard while backing it up with your food intake.

Everyone can build muscle but you have to keep stimulating the body so it sends out a signal to grow new muscle while eating adequately. This is much easier said than done. However, if you are consistent and use the appropriate techniques you will make progress.

You need to have time, dedication and patience to develop your physique. It is akin to gardening where you need persistence to put in the work in and then patience to watch your plants, trees and bushes grow.

Muscle Gaining Myths

Just as you saw in the fat loss section there are also a host of inaccuracies or outright lies when it comes to building muscle. Here are some of the more major ones that you may have comes across –

You Have to Eat Protein Every 3 Hours – This is not true, while practically it may be helpful to spread out the protein consumption you do not have to be eating every 3 hours and carrying your food around in boxes.

You Can Only Absorb 30g of Protein / Meal – If you eat more than this it just takes longer to digest the food and then it gets absorbed. Total protein intake is the main factor to worry about and not how often or when you eat it.

You Need to Eat Chicken, Broccoli and Rice to Gain Muscle – The famous bland bodybuilding diet of tuna, egg whites and chicken with rice and veg is not the only way to make progress. You can grow muscle without any of those foods.

You Must Food Prep for Results – Making thirty boxes of food in one go for the week ahead is not necessary to achieve results. Your body just needs a stimulus to grow muscle and then the food to develop it. The body does not judge you by how many meals you planned ahead, just what you eat.

You Can Lose Your Gains Quickly – This unfounded fear that you can lose muscle quickly is not true. Muscle is slow on, slow off. Only injury or prolonged inactivity will cause losses. This is true even when dieting, losses are less than people suspect if the fat loss plan is sensible. 'Quick losses' normally refer to your loss of pump from a lack of recent training sessions, carb depletion, dehydration and/or fat gain during a period of inactivity. These make you look flat in the mirror.

You Must Use Shakes & Supplements to Gain Muscle– This myth stems from the huge amount of promotion done by the protein and supplement manufacturers. One of the main ways they do this is through their sponsored athletes. Almost every ripped person on social media is sponsored by some sort of company, the majority are probably on steroids but say they are natural. You do not need any supplements or protein shakes to make progress. You may find it convenient and may find some help but you do not have to take them. Even if you did you wouldn't need to do it all year round.

Low Reps / Heavy Weights are the Best for Muscle Gains – The best methodology for growth varies between individuals and everyone should vary their plan, so it is a total waste of time arguing what is the best method. Find what works for you through experimentation. Traditional bodybuilding reaches fatigue within 5 – 15 reps and focuses on the burn.

You have to do Deadlifts or Squats to Gain Muscle – While big lifts may help your hormonal environment there are other options to doing squats or deadlifts. These two exercises can cause injury if done incorrectly or if you have joint issues. You can build muscle with or without them.

No Pain - No Gain – You should never feel pain in any joints at any point when lifting weights. While muscle burn and fatigue is generally good if you are looking to grow muscle it is not completely necessary. The basis of muscle gain is being consistent, therefore you may do some lighter and easier sessions rather than missing a session if not very motivated. On top of that there are various ways to change your approach to still create a stimulus for muscle growth without having to be in lots of pain. The bigger you get or the less time you want to dedicate to training the more you need to rely on high effort training which falls into the no pain-no gain ethos.

You Need Steroids To Get Big – If you have ever been to a natural, drug tested body building show you will know that you do not need steroids to be really big.

You Would Be Pro Bodybuilder If You Used Steroids – Too many people blame their lack of results on being natural and not the fact they do it wrong and/or inconsistently. Taking steroids would no way ensure you get great results let alone become a pro bodybuilder. Also, if you tried to make it in bodybuilding you would have to compete with others who are already taking steroids, then what?

I cannot Build Muscle Because Of my Genetics – Everyone can build muscle, the body has to respond that way if you continue to give it the right stimulus and eat correctly. It is more likely your training is inconsistent and of low intensity. In addition to this you probably do not eat enough food and /or haven't addressed some of the advanced techniques mentioned previously.

You Need a Gym to Grow Muscle – There are plenty of people with great amounts of muscle from training at home, using bars, doing gymnastics and so forth. While it is a convenient way to train, it certainly is not the only way.

You Need to Use a 5 Day Split – The classic 'Bro split' has you training five days a week. Typically you would do chest on day 1, then back, legs, shoulders and finally arms on days 2-5. This covers every body part once per week. You do not need to do a 5 day split, this is just one way to train. Most people do better on shorter splits ideally hitting each body part twice a week.

You Cannot Gain Muscle When Dieting – You can build muscle in a calorie deficit and bodybuilders (without steroids) and people brand new to exercise do it all the time.

Think of it this way, if you need 2000 calories a day to exist and you eat 1800 the body makes up the 200 calorie short fall by using some of your fat reserves (therefore you lose fat over time). If you need say 2050 calories a day to exist and build muscle yet eat 1800 calories, your body can make up this 250 calorie deficit once again using your fat stores and still build muscle. This means you lose fat and build muscle at the same time. This is what body re-composition is all about.

You will of course need to do all the other elements discussed previously to build muscle and your potential to grow is usually less that when eating more food but you can still make progress. This is especially true if you are new to resistance training.

*****

You now know the full mechanics of building muscle. Learning the theory is not that hard, developing the basic skills of lifting is also not so difficult. The challenge comes in developing the more advanced methods and then being able to integrate them into your lifestyle so you remain consistent long term.

How Do You Change Posture

The very final element about changing your physical appearance is posture and creating a flat stomach. Depending on your goals you may need to work on these.

Posture

How you stand or sit has a big influence on how you feel as well as how you look. Your posture is the most comfortable position for your body to take under gravity. In the quest for looking good posture often gets overlooked in comparison to trying to tone up, lose fat or add muscle. However, we are hard wired to interpret posture as it is a big part of body language which we use to evaluate and interpret how someone is acting.

Posture is formed in response to how you sit and stand as well as from the effect of repeated movements in life. It is also influenced by any compensation that occurs from injuries and pains. Almost everyone has adapted their posture to be optimised for sitting down because we spend so much time in that position. The main ways to optimise and change your posture include;

Stretching & Release Techniques –

As a result of holding prolonged positions you will become stiffer in particular areas of the body and have lower muscle integrity (tension, muscle knots etc.). These combine to keep your muscles short or overactive.

To get around this you can use traditional stretching or releases techniques such as massage, fascia release, foam rollers or advanced stretching methods.

The key to this area is to know which muscles to stretch to improve posture. Not all stiff, tight or sore muscles need to be released. Only the short, tight muscles that are distorting posture need releasing. Unfortunately, posture is really complicated. Any simplified generalisation of ideal alignment is probably not actually true for your body. This is because every joint can move in two directions which means you do not know if a muscle is tight or if the joint is out of position.

For example, from prolonged sitting the vast majority of the population's pelvis tilts down (the front is lower than the back). This means that your hamstrings are less in need of stretching compared to your thighs. Yet the vast majority of posture rehab programmes have people stretching mostly the hamstrings. This is inconsistent to the posture most people display.

Strengthening

When a muscle or area of the body is tight then another usually will be weak. Postural correction needs you to strengthen these areas. Once you have identified which muscles need strengthening it can often be difficult to get them to actually work during the exercises. This is because a distorted posture switches them off which allows for further imbalances. You will therefore often need to focus on waking the weak muscle areas up before you can actually strengthen them.

Retraining Neuromuscular patterns

It may be necessary to retrain your brain to remember to use your new postural alignment. This is especially true when looking to maintain certain postural changes during movement.

Countering Daily Postural Imbalances

Very often you will need to instigate a quick routine to counter long term postural stresses, e.g. if you are going to sit down for 12 hours every day then you may need a 5 minute stretch routine to do before, during or after such a long sitting period. This may also include looking at how you sit during the day to reduce some of the impact on your postural imbalances. It is also important to consider your sleep position as we spend such a large part of lives in bed.

Addressing Posture and Using Professionals

If you are a typical posture case then a basic anti sitting posture routine could work very well. However, if you are injured or have numerous pains on the body then you may need professional help in some form.

A simple way to look at posture is through structured programmes like in Pilates and Yoga. Albeit, many commercial versions are too dominant in stretching the back of your body compared to the front. However, it is good to experiment and see how it helps you.

If in doubt around posture it is wise to just focus on your front line flexibility. This means stretching everything on the front of the body and strengthening the muscles on the back.

If you are still having postural issues or pains despite following the above options then you may need to use a professional. This could mean working with an osteopath, chiropractor, masseuse, body work therapist, physio or a personal trainer who is used to dealing with injuries or postural imbalances.

Flat Stomach

A sub set of posture is the stomach area, which is often the worst part of the body for many people. Almost everyone feels they have to lose body fat to get rid of their stomach but sometimes this is not the case, instead the problem is that the stomach is sticking out for reasons other than the fat on top. An example of this is how you may have a flatter stomach in the morning compared to the evening. The only thing that could noticeable change in that time is bloating and digestive issues. So if you want a flat stomach it is about working out what factors you need to address, these could include;

Stomach Activation

Your transverse abdominals act like a corset and are found below the main bigger abs muscles which bend your trunk when doing crunches. Your transverse abs are what most people refer to as 'the core'. They draw your stomach into the spine which protects you back and makes you appear thinner.

It is common for these core muscles to be asleep because they get shut down from eating bad foods or if you have pain in the lower back or pelvis region. When this happens it limits your ability to be able to draw in your lower abs which reduces your potential to have a flat stomach.

The same applies to the oblique muscles which also act like a corset with an influence on your sides. This affects how much you can draw in your waist to appear thinner.

Front Line Flexibility

An issue with having a flat stomach can come simply from being stiff down the front side of the body. When this happens you will be too tight to keep your rib cage high and be able to hold your stomach in. When you are standing with a high rib cage it makes you look smaller through the waist and is deemed good posture. If your front line is too tight you will either stand tall but have your stomach stick out or stand crouched over when your stomach is held in. Both of these positions will not mean you are looking your best.

A tight front line happens from being in prolonged sitting postures. This issue can be resolved by using stretching or other release techniques on the front side of the body. Using stomach vacuum techniques from bodybuilding can also have great benefits when this is a problem.

Bloating

The simplest cause of bloating is from the volume of food or drink in the digestive tract, e.g. if you drink 2 litres of water quickly your stomach will be bloated from the liquid. The same applies to having a big meal. This type of bloating should pass fairly soon.

Other reasons for bloating may stem from eating foods that your digestive system has trouble processing. This can leave you feeling bloated even though you haven't eaten that much. This bloating can last from hours to days. The best way to approach this is to experiment with food elimination protocols to see how certain food groups affect the digestive tract.

The final factor comes from a compromised digestive system itself. These problems can lead to prolonged and significant bloating. When your digestive tract is undermined you may find many different foods will agitate it or create bloating.

This could stem from imbalances in gut bacteria balance or because you picked up a parasite a while ago. To resolve these problems you may need to use large doses of probiotics or protocols to rebuild the gut wall or remove digestive pathogens. This area may need the help of a health professional or a doctor.

Losing Body Fat

While the above factors are important for having a flatter stomach most people also need to lose some body fat to reach their final goal. If you are fairly lean already then this may not be the case. Genuine body fat changes affecting your stomach are slow week to week while the non-body fat influences can be much faster. Whatever your current levels these other factors can make your stomach appear smaller or bigger.

The Practical Approach of Posture Change

For most people they would address this area in addition to their other goals of fat loss or muscle gain. This may involve a small daily stretching routine or adding in posture or stomach activation work at the end of a workout or while watching TV.

Digestion approaches would be introduced alongside any fat loss protocols or perhaps during any maintenance period when you have more mental energy to dedicate to it.

For most aspects of this area you would try a behaviour focused on a small element for a period of time, observe the results and then adjust the plan going forwards.

How Do You Develop Optimal Health

Most people assume that changing your body and developing your health are the same. While they can be similar in process they are different. Developing your health is about increasing energy and improving your health traits, it is about reducing the likelihood of future problems through addressing behaviours known to negatively affect the body. Losing body fat is about consuming less energy than you need. This can be done with or without addressing the areas of health.

While the process of bringing your weight back into the 'normal' range improves your health and likewise when most people eat healthier they usually lose a little bit of weight, there is a big difference between focusing on one of these elements compared to addressing them simultaneously.

In my experience almost everyone can lose body fat and almost everyone can improve their health. However, most people are not able to do both maximally at the same time. This is as much to do with mental energy and time availability as anything else.

Some of the main areas to consider when it comes to developing health include the following;

Optimal Food Intake Amount

There is much confusion around how much food intake is optimal for health because most people only try to optimise their health when also trying to lose weight. The optimal food intake amount for health is the point just before you start gaining body fat. If you need 2500 calories a day then optimal health intake is 2500 calories. It is for this reason why you can never have one nutrition schema that optimises both fat loss and health.

If you need 2500 calories a day, then the optimal fat loss plan would perhaps be 2000 calories while the optimal health plan would be the maintenance amount of 2500 cals. There is no merit to under eating <u>unless</u> you want to lose body fat.

If you want to lose fat and optimise health you will need to account for both aspects. This can be done by rotating between the different calorie thresholds. Albeit you could make an argument that the health benefits of losing fat would offset any negative effects of under eating for a short period.

It is important that you do not overeat when trying to optimise health. Despite what most people believe it is both possible and very common to overeat while eating healthy foods. Many foods that are good for you are also very high in calories, e.g. nuts & oils have more calories than chocolate.

Foods You Eat

The foods you eat give you the opportunity to provide the body with all the vitamins and minerals you need. You would look to optimise these micro-nutrients as well as eating adequate amounts of protein, carbs and fat for efficient energy utilisation.

To hit your micronutrient needs you would need to use a variety of different food sources to obtain the full profile of needed nutritional elements. This can be checked using an app that counts vitamins or failing that as a general guide by having a wide variety of colours and food sources.

It is beneficial to check your micronutrient content of your diet if health is your goal. Simply eating a few green vegetables does not give you the full vitamin profile. This is especially important if you have made any specific eating choices such as going vegan, low carb etc.

Supplements can play an important role here to make up any short falls in nutrients and also to maximise nutrient levels within the body. There are certain nutrients that most people struggle to consume in ideal amounts, e.g. Vitamin D, B12 for vegetarians etc.

Food to Avoid

The other side to eating for health is trying to minimise foods and chemicals that can annoy the body. There are two elements to this, one is reducing toxins found within food and the other is reducing foods known to irritate your body.

The desire to reduce toxins is what created the organic food industry and many cooking or preparation techniques are focused on this element as well. The less chemicals and potentially toxic materials entering your body the better it is for your health. This includes reducing processed foods.

The issue of food irritations can have a huge effect upon your health. A food irritation is any food that annoys your body to some degree. This may be an official food sensitivity involving the immune system e.g. a nut allergy. Alternatively, the foods may agitate the body via a non-immune pathway, e.g. dairy intolerance affecting your gut.

Depending on how you classify food irritations[28] there are at least 4 different types and no test that can show all of them, in fact some types have no test that can identify them at all. The best way to handle food irritations is through structured eliminations during the year and using tests if needed.

The real problem in this area is that the consequences of food irritations are so subtle. Perhaps an agitating food group is reducing your energy by 20%, is causing dry skin, bloating or your frequent runny nose. However, these symptoms will be present most of the time so it is hard to see how it is linked to any specific foods you are eating.

This is compounded by the fact it usually takes at least a few days to weeks to truly see the change in symptoms from eliminating a food irritant. There are also other genuine non-food related reasons why you could have those very same symptoms.

In an ideal world you would eliminate every food group or potential source of food irritant at some point during the year, e.g. 2 weeks no dairy or wheat in January, no nightshades for 14 days in March etc. This allows you to see the specific effect of food groups.

Bad Behaviours

The development of optimal health would also include a long term focus on resolving bad behaviours. This would include addressing alcohol, smoking or recreational drugs. It would also involve reducing stress or stopping things that are bad for your mental health.

Good Behaviours

There are certain behaviours you should develop to maximise your health. This would involve addressing your sleep, which is one of the fundamental bases of good health as well as your breathing patterns. It would also include improving your mental health and happiness. Social contact plays an important role in this category.

Environmental Factors

This looks at trying to reduce the chemical load you are exposed to in life. This can come from many sources such as deodorants, make-up, cleaning products etc. There is also the issue of environmental sensitivities which may affect the body including electro-magnetic energy, mould and air pollution.

Exercise

It has been clearly shown that a regular exercise routine has dramatic improvements in almost every area of health. To receive these benefits it is much easier than you would think and can come from activities than that most people do not even consider as exercise, e.g. walking. Despite the low thresholds, the majority of people are not meeting these needs. If you are reaching your basic movement requirements easily enough then you can get even more health benefits by improving your fitness levels. However, it is important to not chase these extra gains if it puts you off exercise at the expense of achieving the basic easy to get benefits. It is vital you find a way to meet your exercise needs to optimise your health[29].

Other Factors

There are also many other factors not mentioned so far. This would include your stress levels as well as the influence of your mind and emotions upon optimal health development. Other aspects that need more attention than what is usually given to them include social contact and loneliness which has been shown to have a dramatic impact on health, quality of life and life expectancy.

Advanced Protocols

Optimal health may need to make use of various more advanced health protocols. This can range from fasting methods to digestion rebuilding programmes. There are many different avenues to explore here, this is especially important if you have health issues that continue to give you problems despite your efforts in the previous areas. Some of these plans may need to be administered through doctors.

Individuality

It is important to be aware of the issue of how your body is unique. Biochemical individuality[30] refers to how we are the same fundamentally but how we also show great variety between individuals. This shows itself in all sorts of traits from enzyme efficiency to organ size as well as your nutritional needs.

In the real world this means that you may need to eat different foods to the next person to feel satisfied or you may respond better to one exercise plan over another. It could be that you need to prioritise one health element sooner compared to someone else and so forth.

Monitoring Results

One issue with developing your health is the inability to easily chart your progress. In general we evaluate our health based on our energy or if a particular trait is annoying us, e.g. my eczema is playing up. The reality is that the body has a whole host of traits which gives clues into the general state of your current health. The problem is we are not used to noticing them as they are very subtle. Instead we use medical tests to chart progress. However, they often only pick up problems when things have already gone wrong.

The best way around this is to monitor traits that could not be picked up by any medical test. These are called sub-clinical health traits. For example, how often you experience sneezing, dry skin, light headed feeling, poor concentration, low energy and so forth. Through surveying these together you get a snapshot for how the body is doing. By looking at it every few months you can monitor your overall health effectively alongside other measures as used by doctors. This allows you to evaluate the effectiveness of your plan. You can get a copy of my health survey form to complete on my website, go to www.benwilsonuk.com/bonus/

Putting a Functional Plan Together

With so much advice and recommendations it is easy to get intimidated and not know where to start. The problem of addressing health is that there is an almost unlimited amount of things you could do.

The best way around this is to look at your overall levels of behaviours today, then focus on making them a little better by this time next month. There are many ways to start this process. You could cut out a food group, begin exercising, go to bed earlier or add in more vegetables. It depends on your current levels and your desires to change.

Due to the high number of possible actions you could take it is often helpful to have a structured plan on how to approach optimise your health.

The Grand Unified Theory of Weight Loss

How Do You Develop Your Fitness

While a body transformation programme typically changes your fitness it does not have to. You can lose weight by walking and moderating your food intake without ever doing any typical methods of fitness. You can also make significant health gains from exercising at much lower intensities than typically imagined[28]. However, you will perhaps never feel better than when your fitness levels are at a good level.

Fitness can encompass various different elements. It is often associated with the ability to move in aerobic terms such as running, cycling etc. This underpins performance in many sports such as football and benefits general health. For some, fitness refers more to strength training with a big overlap to the muscle gaining process. Another element of fitness is flexibility and coordination as seen within yoga, dance and ballet type movements.

Outside of the health benefits there are two main objectives to fitness. One is being prepared for any fitness pursuit or sport you choose to do. The other is ensuring you have the necessary fitness base to handle all that life has to throw at you. This becomes especially important as you become older. You can still be active and functional whether you are 70, 80 or 90 years of age. You can also improve your fitness levels at any age but the sooner you start the better.

To thrive in general life you will need to be able to squat to pick things off the floor, be fit enough to walk up a hill and have the necessary balance and strength to prevent falls and be free from aches and pains. Whatever your age, goals or desires you should be doing fitness in some form.

Elements to consider when developing fitness include –

Different Stimulus for Different Results –

Fitness can be divided into aerobic, strength and flexibility training. One of the issues in making progress is that each of the attributes needs a completely different stimulus, especially as you get to higher levels within any of them. For example, doing a running programme will not help your strength and lifting weights will not help your running ability. Neither of these will help your flexibility and vice versa.

For general fitness you would be wise to focus on your weaker areas to feel better in the quickest time. If you are really strong but have no aerobic fitness or flexibility you will feel much better if you develop these two elements rather than working on improving your strength yet further. The same would apply to the other areas. The problem is we are creatures of comfort and look to stick to what we are good at doing. However, the best feelings of fitness will come from improving your weak areas.

Fitness Stimulus

Your body does not just develop fitness for no reason. It needs a stimulus to initiate change. This could be you get slightly out of breath going up a hill, you lift a heavy weight while gardening or stretch for five minutes. If you give the body anything that slightly challenges your current fitness abilities it will respond by becoming fitter.

What this stimulus needs to be depends on your current abilities. A new exerciser or 'unfit' person needs to do hardly anything to make progress. A five to 10 minute routine could make great improvements in the early days of fitness training. You would simply need to repeat the stimulus regularly to continue to make progress.

Advancing the Stimulus

As you get fitter you have to give the body a progressively harder challenge to make further improvements. The higher your fitness levels the more advanced methods or techniques you will need to use.

When developing fitness there is a difference between feeling hot, out of breath or sweating vs getting fitter. Just because you are doing exercise it does not mean you are actually improving your fitness. Increasing fitness means you are improving month on month, e.g. you are getting faster, stronger, developing endurance or are more flexible.

The body soon gets bored of doing the same thing. If you have been running for 20 minutes at 10km / hour for months you will not be getting any fitter from this training session. You will get hot and breathe more deeply but your fitness is static, e.g. you are not getting faster nor does it feel any easier.

When the body is on a plateau you need to change the training session to create a new fitness stimulus. There are many different ways to do this. It could be by doing more volume in the session, training more often per week, using higher intensities or more effort. This applies to all areas of fitness from aerobic to strength work. In the previous example you could run for 10 minutes at 12.5 km/h instead of 20 minutes at 10km/h for a month.

To avoid this exercise plateau you need to be changing your training sessions/plan fairly regularly once you have reached a good level of fitness. The fitter you are the more advanced and scientific methods you will need to use. This is shown by the sports science used with professional athletes.

Consistency

The biggest element of fitness development is being consistent over time. All too often the focus with exercise is going hard. However, this is all secondary to being consistent. If you were to jog twice a week for a year, then this time next year you would have done 100 runs and be in an amazing position. It does not matter if runs 5, 16, 17 33 and 67 were pathetically slow. If you keep turning up you will make amazing progress. Some of the sessions will be awful, others amazing. It does not matter if you keep doing your training.

Consistency trumps every other element of fitness. Very often on social media we get impressed by these spectacular workouts and hard core routines. However, what you do not see is those same people doing some very mundane and average sessions which they do not post for us to see. It is impossible to go max out at the same level every session, instead just be consistent and turn up week in week out.

Intensity, Volume & Frequency

The main ways to develop fitness once you have established consistency is through varying the elements of intensity (how hard the exercise is compared to maximum ability) and volume (how much of the exercise you do).

As you get fitter you will eventually run into an issue of frequency as there is only so much energy you can put into any one training session before the body is tired. The only place to go thereafter is to train more frequently and to encompass the advanced method and strategies used within high performance training.

Data

It is very helpful if you use some basic levels of data around your fitness training. When you have some rough numbers to associate to your fitness it is very motivating when you see you are making progress. It also allows you to spot when the body has reached a plateau.

Most people fear taking measurements and the lack of data often ends up ruining your motivation and consistency. If you do not monitor your fitness you will not see how much you improve and miss out on the good feeling that generates.

Performance Variation

A failure to understand the way your body varies in performance can cause you to quit your routine. While actual fitness is slow to develop and even slower to lose, your performance can change massively from day to day for a whole host of reasons.

This means you may run a personal best today and find yourself nowhere near being able to match it in three days' time. You have not lost fitness, it is just your performance was down that day. The fitter you get the less likely you are to be able to perform at personal best levels every session.

Most people get confused by this because of what happens when you first start exercising. When you have low fitness levels you can set a personal best or see improvements almost every session. At higher levels you are lucky to get a personal best once or twice a year. For example, Usain Bolt, the greatest sprinter in history did not set a personal best for the last 8 years of his running career.

It is normal to expect 20% of your sessions to be completely awful and a similar amount to be great. The rest will be somewhere in between. If you are in the process of losing body fat you would expect your bad sessions to be even more frequent due to your reduced food intake.

Variation & Enjoyment

There are so many different types and forms of fitness. While you need to consider which exercise forms are developing aerobic fitness vs strength vs flexibility it usually does not matter so much which you actually choose to do, as long as you have covered all of those bases in some way.

Different exercise forms will have different pros and cons to doing them, e.g. cycling has much less injuries than running but running is much better for bone density. One is not better or worse, they are just different. As you get fitter in any element you will need to be more specific with your choice of exercise and employ more advanced strategies.

As consistency is the biggest factor in exercise performance you must consider your enjoyment in the decision making process of what to do.

Another point to note, do not fall for the thought that you are signing up for life to any exercise routine. All too often people think they have to stick to something once they start. This is not true, if you want to do yoga in winter but play tennis outside in the summer then do it. As long as you stay consistent in some way within the different areas you will make progress, e.g. doing a quick stretch routine after your game of tennis to make up for the missed yoga.

Liking Exercise & Confidence

Many people do not like or feel confident around exercise. This is normal, to improve both of these you need to start off with something that is easy and comfortable and then build your skills. Doing exercise is not mysterious, it is just a skill, like learning to drive or play chess. If you want to learn, you need someone to show you what to do and then you must practice it. With enough repetitions and practice anyone can become confident around exercise.

Improving your enjoyment around exercise is a mixture of developing your knowledge and skills as well as making better decisions on how to do it. Perhaps the main reason people do not like exercise is because they do the same thing for too long so get bored. The next main reason is because they get put off by the effort level and pain of exercising. Neither of these need apply to you and you should work around it.

Becoming consistent with exercise is initially about creating a habit which requires repetitions. The general advice for forming a new habit is that you need somewhere between 21 and 70+ actions to really embed it into your natural routine. In exercise terms this means it will take a few months for it to become natural. This is why you may have struggled with exercise in the past because you were unable to put in the initial amount of sessions to make it a consistent part of your life. An effective plan will account for this process in the earlier days of exercising.

When you have created a habit then consistency becomes king. If you can avoid any long periods of inactivity and missed training sessions during the year you will easily maintain your abilities. To do this the focus needs to be on first just doing the sessions in some form even if it is of low effort /quality.

How to Improve Your Emotional Wellbeing

The mental side of a holistic transformation is fundamental to judging the overall success of any change you make. What is the point of looking a million dollars if you do not feel like it?

As with all of these holistic elements it is assumed that changing your external appearance will bring about a change in the other areas. While that can happen it is not necessarily true. In such cases you will need to do more targeted work. Some of the areas that need specific protocols may include –

Relationship to Eating & Food

It is important to be calm, relaxed and comfortable around food and within your eating behaviours. Irregular eating patterns are very common these days in both terms of overeating and under eating as well as the types of food you choose to eat or avoid.

You should be able to eat any food without guilt, including 'bad' foods. You would want to be free from obsessions and panic about what to eat. At the same time you should be able to naturally balance relaxed or social eating with a healthy eating regime of your own choice.

While changing your body may help your eating patterns it really depends on what method you use to do it. Many diet plans will exacerbate your unwanted eating behaviour rather than help them. It is a fallacy that you need to have good relationship with food to be in shape. Many people with amazing bodies have eating disorders, food obsessions or phobias.

In these situations you would need to address the eating behaviours, patterns and thoughts outside of any transformation plan, either during the process or after you get to your goal.

In many cases it is your poor relationship to food that will stop you achieving your health & fitness goals. In this case you will need to address this area before trying to get in shape.

Improving your behaviour around food may include intuitive eating programmes or specific approaches to address binge eating, healthy eating or your thought process around food.

Body Image

It is assumed that changing your shape will improve / resolve your issues around body image. This is often not the case and you will need to do more targeted work on improving this area independent of any transformation plan.

As with eating behaviours you may find you have to improve body image issues before you are able to get results using typical transformation plans. For example, it may be that until you stop hating your own body you are never patient enough to use a slower more moderate approach to fat loss.

Changes in body image can be done by looking at your thought processes and beliefs in relation to your body. From this you will be able to create a more helpful and supportive structure to use in the future.

Self-Confidence

The process of changing your body is powerful at increasing your self-confidence. This happens from both the changes you create externally and by doing the necessary tasks that create those changes, e.g. exercise, eating a healthy diet etc. Very often however, you will need to do more than just changing your body to truly achieve your desired levels of self-confidence. This can mean developing other skills, doing certain tasks or learning specific knowledge. It could be necessary to examine some events from the past or commit to a project going forwards.

Life Circumstances

While improving and changing your body will positively influence almost every area of your life very often your body transformation was done in a hope to change a specific area, e.g. when I am in shape I will find a perfect partner or my relationship will improve etc.

While it may be true that changing your body improves this other goal it is also common to find that things need to be done in addition to changing your body. This would relate to the specific elements underpinning these other objectives.

Almost any area of your life is based on your focus, habits and actions within that aspect over the last few years. If you change these inputs then you can change and improve that area of your life. This may be your career, social life, love life or more.

*****

Regardless of your specific goals around emotional wellbeing there are certain aspects you will need to consider if looking to improve your outcomes, these include –

Current Beliefs

It is your current beliefs in each of the areas that will serve to lock in your behaviours patterns and/or create resistance to change. The vast majority of your beliefs were not created from choice but you were given them, often from very young. Beliefs are not true per se but they are your perception and interpretation of the world. It is best to look at them in regards to whether they do, or do not serve you. Changing these holistic areas involves looking at your beliefs to see which ones are causing some of your issues and replacing them with more helpful ones.

Current Frames Of Reference

A frame of reference is a system by which you are measuring yourself, either consciously or subconsciously. They are your beliefs made into a process for self-evaluation.

The problem with frames of reference is that they are often inconsistent, dysfunctional or set up so you can never win. If this happens then you will never be able to improve the wellbeing area due to your evaluation process. The goal would be to adjust and develop your frames of reference that would then allow you to succeed and feel good.

Identifying Objectives

Many of the wellbeing goals suffer from a lack of clarity about what you want to achieve. You will usually know what you do not want to have, e.g. I do not want to obsess about food or I'm tired of worrying about how I look naked etc. However, you will often not clarify what you actually want to experience and how that would look in the real world. Creating a positive vision can greatly help the process going forwards.

Defining New Beliefs & Frames Of Reference

With a clear objective it is now easier to identify what beliefs you need to have and the frames of reference to allow you to achieve your goals. This involves consciously creating a more helpful set of beliefs and the basis upon which they are built.

Taking Action

You will need to take action to create change in both your beliefs and any external results. For many ingrained beliefs you will only be able to change them from through doing new behaviours and noticing the results that happen. Action is the key for success in all of these areas of wellbeing. It is very hard to just think yourself out of one set of beliefs and into another. You will need action to facilitate the change.

Creating a Habit

Repeated actions will lead to new habits, which is the end point of behaviour change. This includes not just action based habits but also how your habitual thought processes operate. Real life changes are cemented through repetition. Over time this will create new automated behaviours and thought patterns.

Addressing the Emotional Component

It is frequently the case that improvement in these areas will need you to address the emotional contribution behind it. While redefining beliefs, frames and taking action all serve to change your emotional perspective sometimes you will need to also use emotional management techniques. These methods can be applied to past events, current beliefs or thoughts around certain issues. Changing your connection to these elements can transform your feelings.

Managing Focus & Accepting Limitations

You probably have at least one or two of these holistic goals alongside your desire to transform the body. Most people demand that that they achieve all of these immediately. However, multiple goals usually require different actions and sometimes cannot be achieved simultaneously.

The Cross Benefits of Health & Fitness Efforts

In reality putting effort into one goal will almost always bring a benefit of some sort in another. For example, losing 5kg will improve your running and starting a running programme will probably help you lose weight. When you take any action in one area it has the potential to improve the other areas within your holistic goal.

The Limits of Focus When Achieving Your End Goal

In my experience, almost everyone can lose weight and almost everyone can improve their health, increase fitness or change their emotional wellbeing. However, most people will struggle to do them all at the same time.

As mentioned above, making an improvement in one area will create some improvements in the other. However, it usually takes a different effort and focus to achieve these varying end goals. This makes it harder to achieve all the objectives at the same time.

This is especially true when fat loss is involved. The process of losing weight is a psychological negotiation at times where your body wants you to quit while your mind is split, half of you would like to carry on and the other half wants to stop immediately. The way to self-negotiate these moments is through compromise.

The problem with focusing on two goals simultaneously is that it is very hard to make a compromise that serves both plans. This means you end up trying to follow a regime that is too rigid due to all of your goal demands and eventually you quit everything.

This is a waste and a shame, your failed effort was not because you did not have the skills or motivation to achieve your objectives. It happened because you asked yourself to do too much at the same time.

I always find it strange that in an area where you have struggled to be successful for many years you would be so rigid to demand to lose weight, optimise your health, develop your fitness and redefine your relationship to your body all at the same time. This is what most people do and it simply is asking way too much of yourself.

Rotating the Major Focus

With competing goals demanding your attention they can be balanced by changing the major focus over time. You may focus on one element for two months, followed by a month on another area. This is often done naturally within the body transformation process or can be structured into the plan with use of different phases.

During most transformations you will go through a period of fat loss, followed by a plateau and then a further fat loss period and so on. This is healthy, sensible and what happens in the actual real world of results. On these plateau periods, where you take a break from fat loss, you can put more efforts into one of your other goal areas.

For example, if you want to develop your health and lose weight, you may lose body fat for two months then use a break even month to try some food experiments, e.g. you do a sugar detox and re-connect to natural hunger patterns. In month four you would return to losing weight. At this point you will be more skilled and better at fat loss due to your health focused actions in the previous month.

You may ask, why not do the sugar detox month 1 to lose weight? This comes back to the how much mental energy you have to be able to actually follow the plan. Most people can lose weight and most can follow a sugar detox. Only a few are able to do both at the same time. It is about the odds of success vs effort you can put in.

Accepting Your Limits

The key to all of this is patience. It is the underlying attitude behind achieving all of your health and fitness goals. If you have failed to get results for 2, 5 or 10 years plus then why are you arguing over whether you are at your goal weight by June 10th or July 20th? It is completely insignificant in the big picture if this is the only time you need to do it ever again.

Likewise, if you want to optimise health and to be at your goal weight does it matter if you achieve it by March or September? It would be so fundamentally life changing if you finally attained both you would not care 10 years down the line if it took six months longer to achieve. All too often you will try to achieve your goals too quickly and will not want to compromise your multi goal approach. This is setting you up for failure.

It is helpful to understand you are not giving up on any goals. You do not have to exclude or stop your efforts in one area. Rather, you just need to be prepared for any self-negotiation period where you are struggling with motivation to be open to compromise within one area.

For example, you are demotivated at the thought of a tough gym session and your planned chicken salad this evening so you are thinking about quitting. Instead of trying to push through it you should just accept that today you will not work on your fitness and perhaps just go for a walk. Alternatively, you will do your work out but then be ok with eating something more appealing than the salad. This kind of compromise can keep you in the game. However, having multiple goals can make it hard to make these self-negotiations happen in the moment.

In many of the areas you simply need to work on them while not trying to lose body fat. To address binge eating while under eating (losing body fat) is very very difficult to do. The fat loss process itself is one of the major causes of binge eating. Many changes in health behaviours, e.g. giving up a food, stopping drinking, quitting smoking or trying new behaviours, are many times harder or become impossible to do while also trying to lose body fat.

The Long Game

If you have enough patience and accept you are here for the long game you can easily achieve all of your goals. It should be noted that while some goals like weight loss have a clear end point, other areas such as fitness and health are ongoing. While it is good to have short term goals in all areas there should be no panicked or feel rushed to achieve your aims. Once you have attained your goal body fat you would then focus on these areas as part of your ongoing efforts.

Section 2 – Summary

-**How Physical Change Happens** – Fat loss happens by eating less food than you need over a prolonged period of time. The bigger the calorie deficit the faster the results yet harder it is to follow. You cannot just under eat and not expect your body to fight back to try and make you "fail" on the plan. When you lose fat it will not come from your worst areas initially.

You gain muscle by consistently creating a stimulus for new muscle growth over a prolonged period of time. You have to develop the programme to ensure the body keeps sending out this stimulus. Over the years this requires more time per week and effort per session.

Posture and a flat stomach can be developed by stretching certain tight muscles / areas and strengthening the weaker parts. The stomach area may need a change in diet or protocols to improve digestion to be flatter.

-**How Holistic Goals Are Achieved** – Your health, fitness and emotional wellbeing goals are achieved by using specific protocols for each area.

Health is developed through choosing healthier foods, reducing food irritants, doing exercise, reducing toxins and changing how many good or bad health behaviours you do.

Fitness includes aerobic, strength and flexibility. It is developed through consistently applying a stimulus over time.

Emotional wellbeing goals are developed through addressing your current beliefs, setting objectives and then forming new beliefs through action and emotional management.

Often you will only attain success in multiple goals by adjusting which aspect is your major focus at any one time.

****

Gladys, 65 – For most of her life she was slim and active but after a difficult few years she has gained weight. After retiring five years ago she suffered the loss of her mother and then her husband in fairly quick succession. Further changes happened when her close friend lost her battle to cancer and another moved abroad. With all this upheaval Gladys spent most of her time feeling alone, she had no weight loss goals really as it would not affect her life but she knew it would aid her health and she wanted to feel better.

The conventional approach to changing her body would fail Gladys before it even got started. It is assumes the person wants to change shape and that they have some form of motivation to begin with. She knew she should lose weight but truth be told she did not have any real desire to do it. This meant she would never start a plan or programme.

The changes Gladys made were not from any health or fitness plan but instead from realising she needed to feel happy again. With such a huge change in recent years she decided to address her emotions. She hired a counsellor for weekly sessions and did a course on meditations. She would then do between 10-20 minutes meditating every day. To improve her mood she joined a gym where I met her and also a walking group. For mental stimulation she started classes down at the local college (first a cooking course and then Spanish). She also did some volunteering work with refugees.

It took time but over the months she became more at peace emotionally and developed a nice social network. Without really trying consciously she lost the excess weight because she was active and felt happier. This meant she found it easy to eat sensibly and managed to maintain her results.

****

Section 3

The Grand Unified Theory of Body Transformations

The previous sections have given you a solid foundation upon which you can transform your body. You have learnt the fundamentals for success and all the theory and knowledge you would need to achieve your goals. If everything else was in place then this would already be enough for you to get results. However, for most people knowledge is not enough to consistently take action in the real world.

To do this you need new behaviour patterns, new thoughts and new feelings. You will need to account for who you are as a person and your specific needs to create new behaviour patterns. This must account for your values, your previous experiences and current life circumstances. The Grand Unified Theory of Body Transformations is the process by which this can happen.

In this section you will discover the many different influences upon results and learn which ones may or may not apply to you. You will gain insight into why most people struggle and what factors allow some to go on and be successful with their transformations. This can then be applied to your individual circumstances.

Why A Grand Unified Theory?

If you are like most people then you would have struggled with trying to change your body. Too many people fail too much of the time. This applies within all population groups from young to old and across the world.

The lack of results in general is made worse by the fact there is nothing stopping you or anyone achieving your goals. There are no limits to how many people can succeed. It is not like getting promoted at work, winning the Olympics or building the biggest business in your town. In these cases there is only a limited number of positions available, only one person can win or get promoted. When changing your body literally everyone can succeed as results are about your own actions and it is irrelevant what others are doing.

The Grand Unified Theory of Body Transformations is the collection of answers to the question, what do you need to do to change your body? It accounts for the different needs seen across various individual circumstances. It operates on the level of creating real life and sustained behaviour change. This means that you can get results despite your previous struggles and within your current circumstances

The theory allows you to see the difference between those who obtain great success and those who always fail. It also allows us to look at society as a whole and explain the current situation around body shape.

I created the theory as a natural conclusion of studying how to get results. It is still evolving and adapting to the latest research and hopefully many people will contribute to its development over time.

The Results Process

At the very simplest outlook of getting results there is the following imaginary situation. You are living your life and planning on changing your body. Along comes a food and exercise plan, you follow it and you achieve all you goals. Better than that, you maintain these results forever afterwards. The diagram below sums up the process:

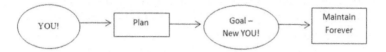

Everyone knows that this is not what happens in the real world 99% of the time yet you probably still approach getting in shape using this schema. As you know, what really happens is you start following your plan and it has to compete with everything else in life. This either immediately stops any progress or slowly wears you down over time.

Even if you get to your goals this way you cannot just switch off and relax. You will have to compete with the ongoing demands that life throws at you. This will challenge your health & fitness behaviours. Maybe you get married, change your job or injure yourself. All of these could send you back to where you began. The diagram below shows this more real life experience of the results process:

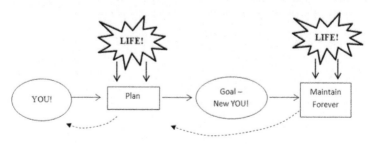

While this schema is better and may appear true, in reality your plan of action and life are not separate entities. They are part and parcel of the same thing. Your plan needs to account for your life and your life needs to include your plan.

It is more sensible to think of there being a balance between positive and negative influences. This would allow us to explain how many people lose weight each year without actually trying. Rather, something changes in their life which alters the balance of positive vs negative influences on their behaviours. This then results in the body changing due to the new helpful actions.

There are various positive and negative influences that can act upon you. Positive ones could include a focused plan of action or trying a new diet, it could be having a clear goal to change your body or maybe spending more time with a friend who is really keen on exercise. Negative influences are all too common, they include stress at work, relationship issues, injuries, health problems, food cravings and more.

The balance of these will determine how much you will progress towards your goals. They will always be competing against each other. One factor that influences the outcome of the balance between the two sides is how many behaviours you do naturally without any conscious effort. For example, if you automatically go and exercise when you are stressed then you will be at a distinct advantage to most people who eat junk food and watch TV under similar situations.

Most plans of action look to implement more positive influences while reducing some negatives ones. The results process could therefore look more like this;

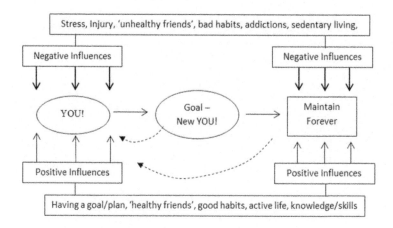

The problem with the above diagram and this way of viewing the process is that it suggests you are going forwards in a linear direction, you become a new you and then maintain this going forwards. This is not quite how life pans out. A better way to look at this is you are in the middle and these processes are happening around you. You are not going anywhere, rather life is influencing you so that you grow and change as a person, including how you look, behave and feel. There are both negative and positive influences and together they will determine the consistency of your actions.

Another element missing from the previous diagram is the duration of your actions. You could have the best day ever or the worst day imaginable, it does not matter if it is only one day. Almost all body transformations of any note take not just weeks but months or perhaps years if trying to build a large amount of muscle. With these adjustments the results process would look more like this;

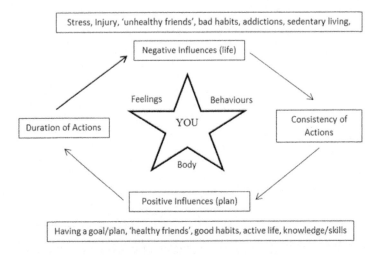

While this schema is perhaps more reflective than the others it is still lacking crucial information. How do we account for the various approaches that have helped people lose weight? So many different methods have benefited people from diet plans to hypnosis and meditation. To factor these in we must separate out the inputs that are known to influence the likelihood of getting results. This would allow us to see along which avenues different approaches work.

This would need to include motivation as well as different types of nutrition & exercise plans. It would have to factor in the influence of our automatic and subconscious behaviour patterns as well. Why do some people naturally do more good or bad behaviours than another? How do you make your desired behaviours become natural? Finally, it must also account for stress, which is one of the most likely reasons for you to fail to stick to any plan or attain results.

It is also important to acknowledge the goal and current position of the individual. How would we approach handling a professional athlete compared to someone who is so overweight they can barely walk? Certain body shapes and transformations will take more time, effort and skill to obtain.

This means any advice and plans needs to be tailored to the appropriate situation and requirement of the individual. Does someone eating take-out meals and junk food seven days a week really need to worry about choosing organic vegetables over non organic? Does a first time exerciser need to follow a 6 day a week bodybuilder programme? This is all about the class of body shape which determines the standard of your needed behaviours. If you factor this into the results process it could be summarised as;

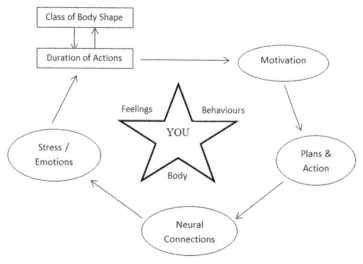

This view of the results process is much better and forms the basis of the unified theory. However, it is still missing certain elements such as the process of choosing to actively change your body and the influence of your identity on your behaviours.

The Grand Unified Theory of Weight Loss

The Grand Unified Theory of Body Transformations

The full and final description of the results process is the Grand Unified Theory of Body Transformations. It is the process by which any one, including you, can achieve your goals. It is not important where you are today, nor do you need to downplay what goals you truly want. You can achieve any goal you desire. To get there though, you will have to develop certain behaviours and these themselves are based off specific thought processes.

The question is <u>not</u> can you achieve your goals? The answer is yes, the question is what process do you need to go through to permanently change your behaviours which would guarantee you go on to achieve your goals?

The body transformation cycle can be seen on the next page. It is the final schema in the discussion about the results process. On first look, it may appear confusing and complicated... Where do you even start? Relax! All of this will become clear as you go through the approach.

The cycle is designed to transform anyone, thus it has many factors to cover all sorts of scenarios. However, you just need to change you. So you do not need to do everything, in fact, it is common that you need to do hardly anything. You may just need to add in one or two new elements from a weaker area.

If you have big goals but they seem very far away, the various elements will give you a clear path on what you need to do. This will work even if no one, including you, believes you can succeed. Results just need you to do the right actions over time. However, remember that the solution is probably not a new diet plan or exercise routine. It will probably be from the various different areas and methods that change behaviour.

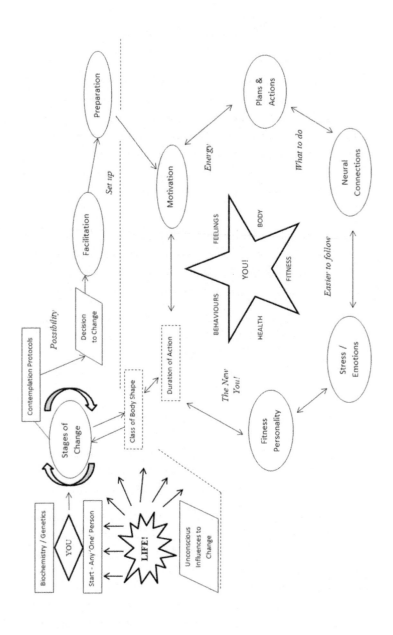

The Transformation Cycle Overview

We will cover each area of the cycle in depth but let's just look at how it fits together and affects results. It starts in the top left corner with YOU.

You vs Life – The cycle begins with you and your life exactly how it is today. This includes the body that you have alongside your thoughts, feeling and behaviours. It also refers to your genetics and current life situation. In addition to this you are being influenced by life as it acts upon you in many ways both positive and negative which impacts your body and behaviours.

Stages of Change – The process of change begins with the steps you must go through to take action. There is the pre-contemplation stage when you are not even considering changing your body which moves into the contemplation stage where you are looking at your options and eventually you get to the point where you decide to make a change.

Facilitation – Upon deciding to take action this stage looks at what programme, approach or method you will use. Many people fail at this exact point before they have even got going by selecting the wrong plan, perhaps the approach doesn't look at behaviour change, they pick the wrong coach or maybe they choose to do it alone when they should have support etc.

Preparation – This phase sets you up for going through the transformation process by putting in place some fundamentals of success. This includes understanding the process of change, looking at when you feel happy about your efforts and ensuring you have an effective measurement system to chart progress.

Motivation – The emphasis is on creating more mental energy to be used during the transformation. It is important to not just focus on starting motivation but on ways of upholding your motivation throughout the process. To do this there are methods to enhance the feelings of your goal, to create a motivating environment and address competing demands upon your attention.

Plans & Actions – This looks at the ABC's of how to change the physical body while allowing for behaviour change. There are nutrition and exercise plans with a focus on sustainability in both the short and the long term. It includes plans for doing the behaviour change elements within the transformation cycle. There are also special protocols for addressing things such as body image, binge eating as well as more advanced protocols. It also includes a focus on simple actions that generate results and how to do these more consistently.

Neural Connections – This area looks at developing and changing your underlying subconscious behaviour patterns and reactions around food, alcohol and exercise. It uses various behaviour change experiments set appropriately for your current abilities.

Stress & Emotions – In this area strategies are used to handle and reduce the influence of stress and negative emotions on your behaviours and efforts. This allows you to still be able to make progress during stressful times.

Fitness Personality – In this part of the cycle the aim is to cement the changes you made to become part of who you are and ensure that you have enough skills and behaviours to achieve your goal. There is a focus on the way you view yourself (your identity), the language you use and the skills, knowledge or beliefs you hold. It also looks at personal growth and the environment around you.

Duration of Action – Body transformations do not happen overnight both physically and behaviour wise. Even if you magically started doing every behaviour perfectly from today forwards it may still take 2, 6 or 12 months plus to arrive at your goal body shape. This is especially true if muscle growth is a big part of your goal. During this stage you would continue to enhance all the previous elements such as motivation, neural connections, stress management etc.

Classes of Body Shape – A body type class represents the amount of skill, effort and time to achieve a certain threshold of body type. It is a generalised classification to ensure you are given the appropriate type of advice needed for your goals. Your class of body changes through the consistent application of needed actions over time.

Back To The Start – YOU/Life & the Stages of Change – After developing into a new body class you return once again to the start of the cycle. You are now a different person to before both inside and out. Your body has changed alongside many of your thoughts, feelings and behaviours. If you have achieved your goal then you would simply ensure that there is a plan in place to maintain results and off-set the negative influences that come from general life.

If you wanted to change your body shape class further you would repeat the whole transformation cycle. This means you would need to go through the contemplation stages until you were ready to take action once more. This time the process would be focus on what is needed for the next body class. This means you would have a different set of behaviours and advice to encompass and focus on achieving.

The Grand Unified Theory of Weight Loss

The Grand Unified Theory in Action

You have already seen a few examples of how the approach can work in the real world with the stories of Kate, Richard & Gladys. There are many more examples:

****

Jane, 34 – She has struggled with weight issues for most of her adult life. She once lost weight doing a Keto diet when she was in her early twenties but not much luck since. She is at home all day with her younger kids and feels stressed. Her relationship with her husband is ok but it is struggling a little. She uses food and a glass of wine (or two) to relax at the end of the day and just to have some pleasure in her life.

A conventional approach would have Jane signing up to some online fitness plan with a low carb keto diet and a short Hiit home workout. She has tried this sort of approach many times despite it never working. Secretly, she knows it will fail before she even begins but she has to do something.

The solution Jane actually used was simple. I told her she could lose weight eating carbs and she reluctantly agreed to test the theory. To her great surprise she not only started to lose fat but she also wasn't hungry. In addition to this she decided she needed to rebuild her social life. She arranged a walk with two mothers she actually liked a few times each week and agreed with her husband to go out with her friends from her last job once a fortnight. None of them had children and kids talk was banned.

After these changes somehow everything was easier to follow. She felt amazing and herself again, like she had her identity back. She lost weight and found it is easy to sustain.

****

****

George, 22 – He has big dreams with his body and wants to be on the cover of a fitness magazine or maybe become a fitness model. He goes to the gym a few times a week but struggles to be consistent as he suffers mental health problems and depression at times. He works in the local supermarket and does not have much disposable income.

The standard route for George would be to go online, follow some of his favourite fitness celebrities and perhaps read an article about what to do. He could download a plan for free or create one from the posts on a bodybuilding forum. He would then go to the gym as best as he could. Using this route George would never achieve his dreams.

The first step he actually took was an acknowledgement. He accepted the requirements for success. He saw how few people achieved this outcome and looked at what they did to get there. He decided to reach out to professional bodybuilders and coaches who train them to ask for advice. He also spoke to me for my opinion. Through these chats he was not just inspired by what he heard but could see how his current actions no way matched his goals. He knew he had to improve his efforts across the board.

He used some money to get a plan and decided to start saving to hire a coach in the future. In the meantime he would train with a couple of guys he knew who were into bodybuilding.

Over time George developed more than just the body he wanted, he changed careers and became a personal trainer. During this process his mental health issues improved so much he barely had a bout of depression. He gained a lot of muscle and started competing in a bodybuilding shows.

****

The Tip of Iceberg

These examples are just a tiny selection of real life stories. You can find similar amongst your friends and social circle. While the credit for many transformations is given to the specific plan almost all genuine success stories have more going on behind the scenes like in the examples.

In the previous scenarios it is easy to swap in other traits that would represent your life more appropriately. Perhaps unlike Jane who is stressed with kids you have been unable to stop eating mostly out of boredom and need to address this.

Rather than being like Richard who is too busy with work and his social life you are without focus after a bad break up and now feel alone. You have dropped into a routine of take outs for one. To turn this around you need motivation and a plan to return to a more enjoyable way of life.

Kate's story would maybe resonate more if she had been obsessed with clean eating but had never exercised. This opposite outlook requires you to relax around food and develop exercise connections.

Where George had to raise his behaviours to be at the appropriate levels for his goals maybe you need to stop trying to use tactics designed for professional bodybuilders. Maybe your plan does not match the needs of your body.

Finally, rather than feeling lonely like Gladys, your main issue might be a vibrant social life which you need to learn how to handle.

What is Your Need?

The above examples show how you have your own needs, circumstances and issues to face and resolve if you want to change your body. You can see how your requirements may be different to what someone else needs to do.

There are many more possible scenarios, situations and problems to overcome that could apply to you or any one individual. At the end of the book I outline a few more specific examples and possible solutions you could use in the troubleshooting section.

Reading about all these scenarios can feel overwhelming because you are reading about many possibilities. In reality, through identifying specifically what you need the process is far simpler and easier than you would have thought.

As you go through the inner workings of the transformation cycle you should be thinking about how it applies to you. No one has access to more information about yourself than you. Make use of it to discover the areas you need to focus upon the most. You can then use this knowledge as you move forwards and apply it to the plans set out later.

*****

Note – Though I appear to criticize the conventional approach of food and exercise plans I am personally behind any change that can inspire long lasting results. There is a definite place amongst the process for conventional plans but they should not be the only approach used and maybe not the best option to use on day one. So if you are following a food or exercise programme you do not need to throw it in the bin, use it as a base to add in the other needed elements on top.

The Transformation Cycle Uncovered

We will now look into the full Grand Unified Theory of Body Transformations by looking at each part of the cycle individually. This will allow you to identify blocks in your current approach and ways to make a breakthrough going forwards.

The cycle can be divided into three main areas, which are the start of the transformation process, the time between deciding to change and taking action and then the core of the transformation cycle itself.

Each of these areas is explained so you can understand how it may influence you to get results going forwards. You will also see the techniques and methods used to create change within each of the areas.

This process is designed to take any one to any goal. It therefore covers many aspects that perhaps do not apply to you directly. Throughout this section be on the look-out for what you feel is applicable. You can also think about other people you know who would benefit from some of the aspects discussed.

The Start of the Transformation Process

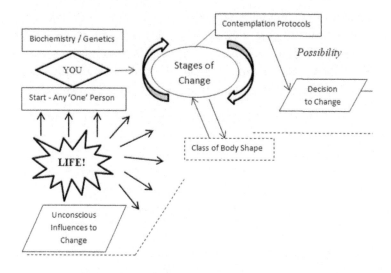

YOU – Any 'One' Person

Before any change has begun or even contemplation of it there is everything you or anyone brings to the start line.

There is no one like you! YOU represents all of your experiences, prior skills and knowledge. This includes your current habits around food, exercise and other areas of life.

YOU includes your body, your age, the genetics you were given, your current biochemistry and more. YOU refers to the strength of your metabolism, enzyme efficiency, gut bacteria profile, hunger, fitness, fat metabolism and much more.

It is not good or bad how you are today, it just is. There is no need to start judging yourself. It is better to just accept and like yourself for exactly how you are right now and then focus on what inspires you going forwards.

Life

Wherever and whoever you may be you will have to deal with what life is throwing at you. This comes in the form of your lifestyle, ongoing stresses, your current habits and the social influences that lock them in place. It includes where you put your mental energy and the things likely to affect this focus.

In general life is pushing you, like most people, in a negative direction around your health & fitness. Without an intervention in some way you are more likely to eat bigger portions and snack more often. We generally become more sedentary as we age rather than becoming more active. Technology creates things to save us from moving rather than making us move more.

With these sorts of influences around you it is important to be slightly on guard about how your body is reacting to just living your normal life.

Class of Body Shape

The combination of YOU vs the influences of life both past and present will determine your class of body shape. This is where you start out on your journey today.

Body shape classes refer to a generalised outcome of body shape based on how much effort, skill, knowledge and time it takes to achieve.

Why Have Classes?

The advantage of categorising body shape is that it means advice can be tailored to you. Perhaps half of the advice given in health & fitness stems from bodybuilding. Hardly anyone wants to be a bodybuilder so why does it influence so much of the advice you follow? This is important as the wrong advice for your needs and goals can ruin adherence and therefore the results you achieve.

Through being able to identify the different goals, behaviours and skill sets needed for a particular result it makes coaching much easier and more efficient. It allows for specific advice and moves away from generalised ideas. It saves you time and effort while getting better results.

The inevitable problems of classes is the moment you separate results into groups then people are quick to jump on it to try show that someone is better or worse than another. This will lead to others twisting their own information to get into a class they perceive as better, or the self-depreciating personalities will undersell themselves to be in a class they perceive as worse.

Classes of body shape are not better or worse than each other! They are representations of how much you need to do and what types of methods you should use. As discussed previously, you decide what goals you want to achieve, it is your body and your life. No one can tell you how your body should be. Wherever your goal may be it will fall into one of the body shape classes which will allow you to know the general behaviours levels needed for results.

Another issue with classes of body shape is that they are robust and general descriptions. This leaves all sorts of room for people to shoot holes in the classification, especially at the edge of one class to another. In the section on Fitness Personality you will see more of the traits within each class.

The Main Class Criteria

The classes are determined in two main ways, one is using your external results as a guide and the other is via actions and behaviour traits. These are;

External Results – This refers to the amount of body fat and muscle mass you have. In general it is harder to have lower levels of body fat and to build higher levels of muscle. This makes it possible to label the different classes of body shape based roughly off these two traits.

Actions & Behaviour Traits – The different body classes also represent how much input is needed to achieve the class of results. This refers to effort, skill, knowledge and duration

Effort is about how much work you must put in, the amount of exercise sessions you need to do, how much meal control or food prep is necessary and how your goals will affect your social life amongst other factors. It also considers your perceived sense of effort, which is how many of the behaviours require conscious focus as they are not automatic.

Skill refers to your ability in the real world to do something. This could be getting yourself to exercise, knowing how to lift weights or being able to cook nice tasting food. It also includes being able to do these behaviours under different emotional conditions such as when you are busy, stressed or feeling down.

There is also the influence of knowledge, which is what underpins many skills. It takes more knowledge to be very low in body fat or have large amounts of muscle. This could be knowledge in the form of what is in food or what your body needs. It would include exercise methods, cooking techniques and the awareness of how to change your motivation and behaviour patterns as outlined in this book.

The final element to consider is the time it takes to achieve your goal. While some people can change body shape class quickly if it is just about losing a little body fat for others it can take many months or longer. When you add in building muscle it may take many years to reach your end goal.

The different classes will have varying demands on how much effort, skill, knowledge or time it will take to achieve a certain standard.

Natural vs Needed Behaviours –

How much of a challenge it is to change body shape refers to how many good behaviours you do naturally vs bad behaviours. If you only ate salad and would go for a run whenever you are stressed, it would be much easier to get in shape than being a typical emotional eater.

A lot of your perceived effort is about how many new behaviours you need to develop. The more behaviours you need to change the harder the challenge and longer it takes to achieve.

The Seven Classes of Body Type

It is possible to separate out the different advice needs and situations into seven classes. These are outlined below. As you learn more on each class think about who you know that fits into each category and where you are on the spectrum.

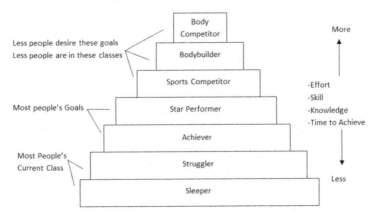

Sleeper – Has no real interest in the issue of getting in shape even if they need to. They rarely or never show any inclination to take action or even consider this whole area.

Struggler – Tries to get into shape but always fails and never seems to progress. Despite all their efforts, diets and fitness plans over the years they are still trying to achieve their goals with limited success.

Achiever – They have managed to be successful with their body. They are in or around the 'normal' body fat range and have achieved a level of results that takes them away from the majority of the population.

Star Performer – They are in the lean, athletic body fat range. They also have an added level of fitness with a base level of muscle from their fitness routines.

Sports Competitor – While being at a lean, healthy body fat like the star performers they have more muscle from their previous training regimes. They may or may not play an actual sport but they are training like they are an athlete.

Bodybuilder – When a sports competitor focuses on just developing their physique they will begin to gain larger amounts of muscle. While still lean body fat wise the extra muscle separates them from the other classes.

Please note that bodybuilding covers various physique goals including bikini fitness, smaller fitness models and other types which are not that classical huge guy look you may associate with the word bodybuilder. This category is someone who is training for a sport, where the sport is building a physique.

Body Competitor – The best of the bodybuilders will look to develop their physique to a standard where they could compete in a fitness model or body building competition. This level is the highest in the pyramid because it takes the most time, skill and dedication to achieve. It is <u>not</u> the most sought after look with it being a more specialised / niche look due to its extreme appearance and requirements.

Body Type Classes & the General Population

Most people are sleepers or strugglers, probably two thirds of the population. Achievers and star performers represent most people's goals. This is a lean, healthy look with a little extra muscle or tone. It can be achieved with fairly sensible demands and is not at all unrealistic.

A percentage of people want more muscle and fall into the other three classes. These classes have less people in them and require more skill, effort, knowledge and time to achieve. Wherever you are today, you can achieve any class with time and dedication.

Stages of change

Without any intervention your body will only change based on the luck of what life throws at you. For the average person that means an increase in weight and decrease in health and fitness. The occasional person will make improvements without trying but life usually has a negative impact on you.

If you decide to intervene in this process then how does that happen and what does it look like? When do you decide to get started? There are two distinct phases to consider;

Pre-Contemplation

In this stage you are not even thinking about changing your body, this could be because you recently failed in an attempt to get in shape, or you have long given up on the possibility of success. Sometimes it is because you have not had the time, space or energy to think about doing anything. It could also be that you do not think there is any point in changing your body. Eventually something will stimulate you to move into the contemplation stage. Perhaps a pair of trousers do not fit, maybe you realise your next birthday is six months away or you start believing it is possible for you to change your body.

Contemplation –

In this stage you are aware that you want to change your body and achieve some sort of goal. Despite this you are not yet at the stage of taking action. This stage can be very short, maybe you see the number on the weighing scales and the diet starts 10 seconds later. For many people though they can spend a fairly long time in this stage. This can be especially true if you do not really know what to do to get results or the options available to you seem rather unappealing.

Factors that go into the process of change

There is no set process to go through the stages of change. However, it would need to include some of the following;

Increase in Belief – You are not going to take much action if you do not feel you can change or that it is impossible to get results. So the contemplation process needs to increase your belief in the possibility of getting results.

Reduction of Perceived Pain – It is common that you avoid committing to your goals because you focus on the negative aspects of what to do and the pain or discomfort it would involve. This needs to be reduced to make change more appealing

Increase in Emotion – This is the fuel by which we take action. To increase emotion you can focus on the current pain of your situation or impending problems that will happen if you do not do something soon. Pain is generally better to get you to start a plan than inspiration around the benefits of the goal. If you do both at the same time then it is much more likely you will commit to an approach.

Increase Urgency – It is common for people to get stuck in the stages of change for ages. Creating a sense of urgency is sometimes necessary to accelerate the decision process.

Social Influence – Other people, be it friends or society at large can be a way to facilitate change. Alternatively, other people can stop it from ever happening. It is helpful to make use of other people as social proof to motivate you into taking action while diminishing any negative impact from certain individuals or groups.

To use this to get started you could think about your previous successes while focusing on the enjoyable aspects you used on that plan. You could then spend some time thinking about how you could start today without the worst bits that are putting you off. Look to visualise the discomfort you currently experiencing because you are not at your goal and then think about the glory of being successful. Finally, book a holiday with a friend to create motivation to start your plan ASAP.

If you wanted to get a friend to become healthier maybe you should start by showing them how success in one area of their life is similar to what is needed in this area. Then explain how they do not need to do any of the bad things they are imagining (being hungry, never eating nice food again etc.) Finally you could remind them of their upcoming birthday and explain you will take them to their first exercise session. This would increase the odds as best you could but even then it may take weeks to months before they took action.

I feel this area is an open to a lot more future research. Marketing models have very advanced processes[31] and I feel those techniques could develop a methodology here. There is not that much difference between trying to sell a product to someone and trying convince yourself to improve your own health.

Decision to Change

The end of the contemplation phase is when you make the actual decision to change. A few points around this;

Decide To Change Before Working Out The Details – There is a difference between committing to do something about your body and working out the exact details of how to do it. The first step is simply acknowledging if you want to change. The next stage (facilitation) will worry about working out the details of how to do it.

The Time to Change – There is almost never a better time to make a decision to change than right here, right now. As time goes on you develop worse behaviours, encounter new stresses and get more out of shape. There will always be this reason or that why it is better to delay focusing on your goals. However, come that time there will be another excuse, then another. Now is the best time to change, it always will be.

Starting Slow – There is no reason to start off in a crazy obsessed way and turn your life on its head. You do not need to throw out all of your bad foods or do a 2 hour exercise session. The hard core approach gets all the attention but the vast majority of people do better starting off slow. An intense approach will often stop you committing to change as it appears so hard. Your decision to change simply means you will look into what the best route forwards could be.

Avoid Infinites & Future Commitment – A major cause of the delay between making a decision to change and actually taking action is thinking you have to do things forever or for a very long time, e.g. I will never eat chocolate again or I will do this boot camp three times a week for a year. You should not plan the details of getting results at this stage anyhow but you should especially avoid considering long term commitments.

Public Knowledge – In the same way that you do not have to start off hard unless you want to you also do not need to tell anyone about your efforts. It is quite possible to start and make progress without anyone really knowing. There are pros and cons to telling others, decide what is best for you. Sometimes the fear of other people knowing that you are trying to get in shape stops you from taking action.

Explaining Your Decision – Just because people may know you are getting into shape you do not need to explain, justify or debate what or why you are doing anything. Often it is the thought of explaining to a specific person why you are doing something that is putting you off deciding to take action. You do not need to explain anything to anyone.

Taking Action & Avoiding Procrastination

After deciding you must change there is this very important step where you consider how you will structure your approach to getting results. So many people can get stuck here, often for many weeks to months or even years. It is important to pick the right actions to get started ASAP yet in a way that sets you up for success.

This stage has a big influence on the likelihood of being successful even though you haven't even started yet! In the vast majority of cases where you fail it could have been predicted on day 1 way before you ever got going. This is due to bad planning or not having the key fundamentals in place. This issue is resolved through the stages of facilitation and preparation.

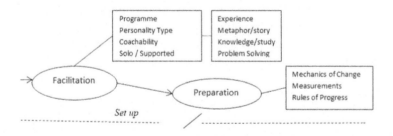

Facilitation

This stage is about weighing up what methods to use and what you will need to be successful. The main things to consider at this point are;

How Will Change Happen?

What will really create change is not just a good plan involving food and exercise but one that focuses on creating new behaviours and developing your skills. You need a plan that encompasses your individual circumstances so that you can actually get results today and in a way you can sustain them long term.

Programmes, Coaches & Doing it Alone

There are no right or wrong ways for change to happen, many people achieve success on their own and many get great results while working with someone or within a programme. The right way depends on your personal situation, finances, personality type and learning style. Transformations are journeys and this will usually involve periods on your own and under the guise of different programmes, coaches or role models. If your progress stalls it is usually a good idea to use a new approach, programme or coach.

Personality Type

There is great diversity in the personality of any two people and making use of this could be a way to accelerate results. Many systems have tried to categorise personality types, there is the 'Big Five' that psychology seems to favour, the very popular Myers Briggs, you have enneagram typing, the LAB profile system and much more[32].

I think this is a big area for potential improvements in results and research should be focused on looking for links between personality type, actions taken and results. I have a feeling that it may come down to traits other than just the ones in the main tests above. For example, the most effective way you are able to learn, your response to coaching etc.

It is also good to make use of your past experiences. What did you enjoy before and what has actually worked for you? Some people go into change at 100 mile an hour to only find they soon quit afterwards, others are slower to start and never quite build any momentum. What can you learn from your past? Use this information you can make wiser and more informed decisions this time round.

Methods of learning

This refers to the different ways you can acquire knowledge;

Experience – What we go through and experience is perhaps the best way to learn. This is especially true within health & fitness. I could tell you how most of your hunger is an illusion and that it will go away within 10 minutes. However, this means nothing compared to when you feel this phenomenon in real life. You can watch exercises videos or read a book on meditation but you need to participate in them to truly experience how they benefit you.

Problem Solving – The time, attention and perhaps frustration you give to solving a problem is one of the best ways to learn. The health & fitness industry is expert/guru lead. So almost by definition you never try to solve your own problems, you are told the answer (which is usually just one answer amongst many). This denies you the benefits of the putting your mind towards the solution and the quality learning that comes with it.

Metaphor / Story – We learn so much through story and metaphor because our brains are hard wired for it. This is why TV, books and films dominate our spare time. While weight loss traditionally falls back to facts you would probably learn much faster through listening to a story that shows the principles of those facts. An easy way to do this is to hear stories of others who have already been successful in changing their body. I feel future research should look to build on this trait further to influence behaviour change.

Knowledge Learning / Study – There are still many merits to the more traditional style of learning but the process of changing your body is heavily influenced by the other methods. Almost all factual knowledge you acquire will also need to be linked to how that feels when applied to actions in the real world.

It is also possible to make the factual learning process into an experience much of the time, e.g. if you want to learn the calorie content of food you could sit there and read a boring book or simply spend a couple of days monitoring your food.

Using the Different Learning Styles

An effective plan will focus on all these methods of learning. The traditional approach is usually factual knowledge based. You are given a plan to learn and follow. If you have a problem you will usually ask for a solution rather than trying to solve it on your own.

To incorporate the different learning styles any plan you use should encourage you to tune into the reactions of your body. Ideally it will also create a variety of situations for you to go through different experiences. This will allow you to learn how certain aspects feel within the body.

In addition to this you would look to try to solve your own problems before asking for help. Coaches should discuss and guide you around your proposed solution rather than telling you what to do before you have had a chance to think about it. You can get access to stories from listening to other peoples experiences. Factual learning is usually done when starting a new plan or trying something new.

*****

In section 4 there are different approaches set out for you to follow which includes and accounts for the above factors. Use one of these easy to follow plans to avoid procrastinating once you have made the decision to change.

Coachability

This refers to how easy you are to be coached, how open you are to doing what is asked of you and receiving honest feedback. This is important even if you are doing this alone. You need to be open to coaching, albeit the coach will be you!

The average person is pretty awful at being coached and does only a small percentage of what is asked. Low coachability shows itself with fights over every detail, a lack of honesty about behaviours, heavy resistance to change and rarely asking for help when struggling. Being coachable is not about being successful with your actions. It is about effort, communication, persistence and working within the process.

Your level of coachability is affected by your personality, prior experience, level of engagement and trust in the process. There is also an element of timing to this. A particular programme may be good enough to get results but you are not in the right head space to get it to work at that particular time of your life. Overall, coachable people get much better results.

Preparation

Even if you have followed the facilitation process correctly it is common for people to fail before they have done their first action. This is due to not having the fundamentals in place.

There are three main areas to consider. If you have them in place already then great stuff, if not, you will need to begin working on them. In either case, this is a process rather than a one off step. As you go through the whole journey these need to remain in place, if they fall below the needed levels then you will need to refocus upon them.

Mechanics of Change

An agreement upon the underlying mechanism of physical changes is vital, especially in fat loss. A large percentage of very motivated people with a balanced and successful mind set fail because they did not grasp the fat loss process. For example, they follow a low carb diet yet their body wants carbs or they are following a huge calorie deficit before inevitably quitting the plan. Almost no motivational technique will help in situations where there are strong nutritional craving from a bad plan.

A fairly good understanding of the mechanics of fat loss is therefore needed. You have already read about this in section two. Understanding the mechanics is best done through experience by actually seeing and feeling these processes work within you. When you have real life experiences and results you will be able to override any contradictory arguments from books and experts as well as challenging your own rigid beliefs.

There needs to also be an understanding of the process by which change can happen in your behaviours, thoughts and feelings. Perhaps the fundamental belief to understand is simply that you can change, which is a block to most people ever trying. This would accompany an understanding that beliefs and thoughts need a different approach to develop them compared to changing physical traits.

Rules of Progress

This refers to the set of rules you have about when you feel good in regards to your efforts. It links into the dopamine system and it is based on the perception of whether you are progressing in the right direction to achieve your goals. This is important because it is a tool to accelerate behaviour change.

Dopamine is a chemical that makes us feel great and it is triggered by many different things such as nice tasting food, social contact or exercise. However, it was originally intended to be used as a reward for making progress on a goal. In the olden days this may have been finding food or shelter. The good feeling you would get on finding these would encourage you to repeat more of the same actions.

To make use of dopamine you need to ensure you have a set of expectations that help to trigger it regularly during the transformation process and not just on achieving the end goal. If the only way you can feel good for your efforts is on that one day you finally achieve your goal you are doomed for failure.

There are three beliefs / rules you should look to encompass into your mind set to capitalize on this reward mechanism. These are outlined below;

Belief 1 - If I Make Any Effort to Get in Shape or Change Behaviour I am Progressing

You should feel great when you try to do anything, especially anything new as this is progress towards your goals. It is not the outcome of your actions that matters but the mere fact you took an action. Repeated actions will help you achieve your goal eventually. The positive emotion you experience from taking action will help accelerate the habit formation process so that you will do it again.

Avoid comparisons to what you didn't do, how much more you could have done or how you could have improved what you did do. If you are trying, you are winning, so this is something to feel good about. Celebrate that you tried!

Belief 2 - If I see Any Positive Results or Changes I am Progressing

Long term success is about being a little bit better today than you were yesterday. So any signs of improvement, however slight, are a step towards goal attainment and that you are on the right path. So this is progress!

It is vital you feel good whenever you make a little progress. This applies to your external results of course but also to your behaviours, internal thoughts or emotions. When you improve in any aspect then feel good about it.

Avoid comparing yourself to where you used to be years ago or where you would like to be in time to come. Do not compare yourself to what other people did or would have done in your situation. Enjoy the feeling of being a bit better today than yesterday.

Belief 3 - If I Make a Mistake I am Kind & Forgiving to Myself as I am Still Progressing

There is no reason to hate yourself for how you are today or chastise yourself for any errors you made, or will make going forwards. This is part of the process.

It is expected that thing will go wrong during a transformation and there is no reason to feel bad about it. Instead feel positive that you are trying and that you keep going even after making mistakes.

Mistakes mean you are trying, mistakes mean you are in the game. If you keep making mistakes eventually you will achieve your goal. So celebrate each one, be kind upon yourself and understand you are still progressing.

*****

When this area is working well your perception of progress is linked to your efforts and not your overall external outcomes. This means you can feel good for trying which results in you doing more and more things. As action creates results, the more you do, the better your results. This means you get further rewards now that you can see progress which fuels yet more behaviours.

The opposite of this is what most people do. You only feel good when you can clearly see you have made an improvement. This means at best you could only feel good every few days and as most people are awful at seeing results it is more likely every few weeks. This gives you no positive feelings, which makes the whole process harder so you end up taking less action which produces even less results. In addition to this, you will want to feel good so you use other methods to get a quick hit, which often involves eating higher calorie foods which disrupts results yet further.

To start making use of these more helpful rules of progress you first need to decide that you want to embrace them. You will then need to make a conscious effort to act in accordance to the rules. When I work with clients it is easier in that I can tell them when to feel good and thus reinforce these patterns.

If you are on your own then it takes a greater responsibility and focus on your behalf. You can explain what you are doing to a friend or partner who could then remind you about your new rules. It can also help if you review your efforts at the day and consciously practice using these methods.

If you get this area right it allows you to experience positive emotion today and every day based on your actions, this is much more productive than having to wait months or years to feel good based on future results.

If you really struggle with this area then it means one of your core beliefs is interfering with these aspects, e.g. beliefs about perfectionism. This can be examined and a more helpful viewpoint can be created. You can get results without a supportive set of rules around progress but you have made it harder for yourself from the very first day.

Measurements & Progress

The final area where most people come unstuck is through their inability to measure, chart and acknowledge progress within the body. This is a real problem and stops so many attempts to get in shape. The transformation can be simplified down to this simple process –

Follow a Plan – Review Results – Continue or Adjust the Plan

The ability to review results is the key to this process. If you have achieved results then you would continue without changing anything. If you have not progressed as desired, then something needs to be adjusted or improved.

However, it is a major problem if you cannot accurately judge progress. If you have you have lost body fat, improved fitness or changed your eating patterns yet you feel you are exactly the same as before then the consequences are huge. There is the initial demotivation of not seeing results but you have also taught yourself that you need an even bigger effort than already given just to get some sort of improvement. This makes the whole process appear unachievable and leads to you quitting.

I have consistently seen clients be unable to spot losses of 2-3% body fat in the first few weeks of training (~1-2kg). As an objective viewer I can easily see they have lost fat yet they cannot. This undermines the results process. They are losing body fat very quickly (around 1% fat per week) yet cannot see it. At that speed they would have made a dramatic transformation within three months and many would have reached their end goal. However, due to being unable to notice or acknowledge results most will quit because 'it is not working' or make it too hard to follow by changing the plan.

To help you with your ability to see progress look to make use of the following elements;

More Than One Measurement – You should never be relying on one method to deliver your results evaluation. What if the measure is inaccurate that day? Unfortunately every measurement method has some issues and drawbacks to using it. Therefore having a selection is far more effective.

Ideally you would use specific items of clothes as your main measure, with circumferences, body fat % and photos as the next best options. In addition to this you could use any of the following but they all bring with it huge potential for errors, this includes the feel of your body, weight, personal evaluation and the thoughts of other people.

Through having four measures of body fat progress over one you are much more able to make sensible evaluations. If you are down in three out four it is clear you have made progress.

Appropriate Timescales – You also need to know when you should be remeasuring. In general, once a week is ok for some measures like clothes but others need a longer period to notice changes. In addition, you need be aware of how measurements affect your motivation to find the most effective strategy for you.

Forget the Weighing Scales – For most people the very worst measure to use is their weight. It carries too much emotional significance and meaning. It is also notoriously bad at reflecting actual body fat changes. Your weight can naturally change between 0.5 to 2kg+ per day simply from what you ate, whether you have gone to the toilet, hydration levels and carb reserves. In addition to this, anyone has the potential to shift their weight by at least 5kg+ through manipulating these factors either accidently (you had a big binge) or on purpose (a 70kg boxer will dehydrate by 5kg to fight weight)

Be Careful With Expectations – Often you will evaluate your success based on how much progress you made vs the expected speed of progress. This can leave you feeling down even though you have improved. This is because you were expecting more results. While it is can be good to get feedback it is not helpful if your expectations are way off or completely unrealistic in the first place.

Remember Your Rules of Progress – It is helpful to ask, why are you measuring yourself? The only reason to measure is to check your progress to evaluate the effectiveness of your plan and adherence towards it. In this sense it should be done in a neutral mood with neutral feelings whatever the results.

Measurements should <u>not</u> be motivational devices. You should not be measuring yourself as a source of motivation. It is a very ineffective strategy. While it is fine if you have made better than expected progress, most times you will probably demotivate yourself. Alternatively, you will only ever remeasure when you are 100% sure you have made progress. This takes away from the overall point of measuring, which is feedback on the effectiveness/adherence to the plan.

If looking for motivation, it should be coming daily from feeling good about your efforts or from the methods you will learn later on. Your measurements should not be a fundamental source of motivation as you will be unable to tap into it most of the time. Measurements and motivation are like flipping a coin, sometimes you win, but half the time you lose. For me those odds are not good enough to be using it in a transformation.

*****

Becoming better at using measurements takes some focus. It is often helped by having a neutral independent person to guide you, e.g. a trainer, your friend or partner.

The Grand Unified Theory of Weight Loss

The Core of the Transformation Cycle

After deciding to change and completing the preparation steps everything is set up for you to enter the core of the transformation cycle and begin transforming your body.

This part of the process is cyclic where all areas are working simultaneously and not step wise where you do one area followed by another. The different influences affect each other as they are synergistic. For example, your motivation affects how you handle stress and your stress affects your motivation.

You do not need to address all areas at the same time. For practical reasons you may just pick one or two areas to begin and then bring in the other influences over time. The more you know what you specifically need to get results the easier it will be to pick an area for the best return on your investment.

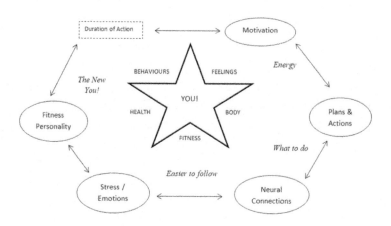

You – A Holistic View

At the centre of the transformation cycle is YOU! Who will experience the effects of the methods used in each area as well as the ongoing influences that comes from living life.

It is useful to remind yourself that a holistic transformation is focused on various elements within YOU and not just your body. This includes your feelings, thoughts, behaviours, your fitness and health. It may well be that some of these other holistic goals are actually higher in priority than changing your body shape.

Throughout the process you should keep an eye on all of these elements. It is not just about how your body is changing but also these other areas. How are they going during the process? It is important to not sacrifice these in the quest for fast results.

The holistic goal elements of developing your health, fitness and emotional wellbeing also need to be considered in regards to how much you can commit to these different goal outcomes at the same time. You should manage your efforts appropriately based off real world feedback. While making progress in any one area usually improves the other, you will need patience to navigate multiple goals. However, with time and an effective plan you can achieve all of your different objectives

Motivation

This part of the body transformation cycle is designed to raise the level of desire you have for your goal and increase the energy you have to put into achieving it. The more motivation you have the better, this also includes willpower which is an aspect of motivation and the terms can almost be used interchangeably.

Motivation is a crucial piece to the puzzle because you have to take action to create new habits. Without some level of motivation this will simply never happen. In general, the higher your motivation, the better your chances of great results. The key though is how you choose to direct your actions when motivated. Sadly, most people misdirect their focus towards short term results and not long term change.

While motivation is important of course it still gets a little too much credit and blame for the level of results achieved. There are many other influences on your results that include your beliefs, values, habits, knowledge, neural pathways and much more.

You would have no doubt tried or seen all sorts of motivational techniques, from your weekly weigh-in to pinning a photo of your next holiday on the wall. Maybe you hired a trainer or put an item of clothing on your cupboard door. While these can be effective there is so much more you can do. In general motivation is a fairly misunderstood area. The following pages should clarify the different elements to it.

Understanding Motivation

There are various elements to motivation some of which you will be familiar with while others will perhaps be new.

Goal vs Task Motivation

Goal Motivation is the classical view of motivation. It is how much you want to achieve your goal and how much better your life would be if you achieved it.

Task Motivation is the desire to do the micro-behaviours your goal requires you to do to be successful. It is your affinity to do the tasks that your goal demands, e.g. how much do you enjoy exercise, cooking, eating healthy food etc.

The greater your motivation in one element the less you need motivation in the other. For example, if you are 100% obsessed with your goal you will do any necessary behaviour even if you do not like doing it, you would just suffer through. Conversely, if you simply love doing the needed micro behaviours, e.g. hitting your step goal, eating small portions, exercising etc. You would achieve your goal body as a side effect of doing the tasks you enjoy without any big lofty goal.

The opposite end of this spectrum is probably more familiar to you. If you have almost no motivation to achieve your overall goal you rarely find the effort to do the needed micro behaviours even if you quite like doing them. Likewise, if you hate all the micro behaviours that are needed to achieve your goal then you will struggle take any action even if you are quite motivated to achieve your overall goal.

For best results you would want to experience your goal motivation more frequently and in greater magnitudes while simultaneously increasing your desire to do any needed micro behaviours.

The Two Ends of Motivation

There are two fundamental drives to motivation. One is that you want to get to an objective and achieve something that excites you, which would bring joy, happiness or other good things. The other is that you are looking to get away from a bad place or experience, you are focused on moving away from pain and ensuring bad things will not happen to you. This was discussed in section 1 in recognising your feelings around change.

The two ends show itself as the carrot or the stick debate. It is whether you use encouraging or berating motivation methods. It is whether you teach people through love and passion or fear and consequence.

In terms of getting in shape it is important that you attune to which end motivates you to take action. You will not be a carrot or the stick motivation type on every aspect. It will vary depending on what you are looking for motivation to do, e.g. go to the gym or resist a food craving. You will get better results if you use the right motivational style in the right places.

Variation of Motivation

Motivation is not a constant thing and there is a difference between peak motivation and persistent motivation. The latter of which is much more influential on your results.

Motivation naturally flows in waves, so at certain points you are feeling more motivated than at other stages, be it within the day, week or over a month. This is the unavoidable reality of how motivation works.

Many people feel that they have something wrong with them if they are not always feeling motivated but this is unrealistic and even top athletes suffer the same issues. The wavelike nature of motivation still allows for you to have a much higher or lower motivation than another person but both of you will experience ups and downs within your own ranges.

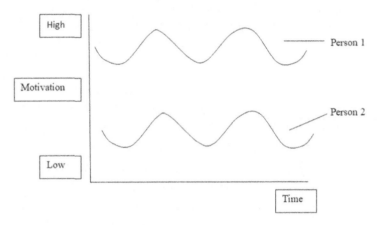

Many things affect the contrasting up and down nature of motivation. A big influencer is overall food intake, when you under eat and lose body fat for extended periods of time your motivation levels will have a gradual decline with periods of lower motivation predominating over higher periods. This means you will need to work harder to maintain motivation as you progress. If you are seeing results then this can often offset these issues. This was discussed in 'Your metabolism as a wave' in section 2.

Other factors that influence motivation include sleep, emotional stress, a busy lifestyle, other people, food, exercise and much more.

Motivation vs The Feeling of Being in Shape

When most people speak about motivation they are often remembering back to a feeling they experienced. This was the emotional high of being in shape or transforming the body. A time when you were focused on your goals and making progress. This is not a motivation feeling per se, this is the feeling of being in shape!

It is a combination of feeling healthy, happy and energised while sticking to your plan and progressing. This motivation feeling comes after the body has begun to respond to a plan. Expecting to feel this way on day one is therefore not a sensible idea as you will need to wait until results have started to happen. Early stage motivation is more of a low key feeling and drive rather than these emotional highs. It is helpful if you have set your expectation appropriately.

The Reality of Motivation

Alongside confusing motivation for just being in shape there is still the belief that being motivated is always about feeling pumped and high. You imagine your fitness efforts to be a scene from a 'Rocky' film. You hope to be firing on all cylinders every day, loving the process while looking and feeling great. This is not at all reflective of the real world of motivation.

Motivation is the inclination to take action towards a goal or a specific task. It can be done as much out of anger as it can joy, or out of necessity as much as choice. To get results it is important you know that you will have periods of average to low motivation in which you do not feel great nor can you give your very best effort.

In these moments it is about keeping going and finding a way to do something in some form. You grind through, one step after another without looking too far ahead. Before long, the difficult period will pass and you will be motivated once more.

This is real life motivation, it is often not pretty but it works. When you do this other people will say you have an underlying drive. This is your true motivational aim, to be someone who is driven.

So spend time considering how to keep going when you are feeling a little flat, this is far more productive than hoping to feel pumped all the time.

Handling Your Waves of Motivation

When you are experiencing a period of high motivation you have a great chance to direct this energy into the other parts of the programme. The biggest mistake you can make is to just use this motivation to follow your conventional plan of action with more intensity. This only works if you already have everything else in place. It is more effective to direct your energy towards methods that fundamentally change how you act within health & fitness as discussed in the other areas of transformation cycle.

In periods of low motivation you need to learn how to edge yourself out of this state. This is about becoming aware of how you are feeling and self-negotiating a way to take the smallest of actions that you are prepared to actually do. Once you have done that action you would then repeat this process. This allows you to nudge yourself back into a more motivated state. Eventually you will feel good and be focused once more. This is one of the fundamental skills around getting results as you will always have periods of low motivation. The quicker you can get out of it the better.

The Four Areas of Motivation

When it comes to using different motivational techniques at a practical level there are four main areas. For optimal results you would want to use all of these at some point during the transformation process.

Goal Emotion

This refers to the level of emotion and desire you have around achieving your goal and making a change. This includes both the magnitude of the emotion and the frequency by which it is experienced.

The emotion you feel will be linked to the quality of your imagery around your goal. This does not have to involve a visual image per se, you can experience emotion from feelings within the body, sounds, words in your head and even smells. The emotion can be positive towards your goal (desire to succeed) and/or negative away from an outcome (fear of the consequences of not changing).

If you are successful in any area of your life there will already be ingrained imagery that creates motivation and drive. If you struggle in any goal area, this imagery will most likely not be imprinted in your emotions or mind.

Frequency is often underestimated when emotion and motivation are discussed. It is better to be slightly motivated at the thought of your goal every day than massively psyched up once a month.

You will want to link any emotion you experience around your goal directly to taking action and doing the key behaviours that produce results. At this point the more you access your goal motivation the more likely you will do the actions that bring results.

Goal Priority

This looks at how much attention is given to your different goals and how they are handled in the face of competing demands. It is common for you to be fairly motivated around your body goals but just find they get swamped by all the other influences upon your time and focus.

You would want to increase the priority of your transformation goals so that they are less easily pushed down the priority order when life gets busy. This can be done by looking at your values and the influence your goal has upon the other areas that currently win your attention. This means you will become better at balancing your goals.

Often people get confused between priority and time demands. Priority means at what point is the area considered or thought about, this is not the same as the amount of time dedicated to it. Very often in health and fitness it takes just a few minutes of attention to get things on track. Work, social and other elements of your life will always have the largest time share. The key is that you consider your needs in this area before you get overrun by everyday living.

Goal priority also includes the influence of task motivation around doing the micro-behaviours. The more appealing they are the easier it is for them to rise in the priority rankings compared to less desirable tasks.

You can often make subtle changes to increase your desire to do the micro behaviours or a specific task. You will want to make any necessary behaviour more appealing.

Goal Environment

This is the situation around you and how it influences your behaviours. A large part of how you act has nothing to do with you and instead depends upon your environment. For example, imagine how you would behave if you were living in a house of Olympic athletes as they prepared for competition compared to living in a house of obese, exercise hating, TV addicts? It is guaranteed you would eat better and do more movement living with the athletes.

While it is not necessary to move house there are various methods you can use which creates a more motivating environment to support you. This can include making use of challenges, groups, external data, trained professionals and much more.

You can think of your environment as a suggestion of how you should act. For example, eating your meals using small plates or leaving your exercise clothes in an obvious place are suggestions to eat smaller portions or go for a run. It is about surrounding yourself with as many of these persuading elements as possible.

When you have these in place you will probably be surprised by how you feel and act. The same old you, will somehow not be acting in the same old ways. Your goal would be to develop a more supportive and motivating environment around you so you do not need to rely on self-motivation all of the time.

Goal Motivation States (Mood States)

This refers to a short term and temporary state of how you feel. There are various mood states that you will cycle in and out of within your everyday living, e.g. a good or bad mood, feeling relaxed or excited, being motivated or demotivated.

These feeling states are encoded in your body through a combination of posture, breathing patterns, the thoughts you focus on, the words you say to yourself and other elements of physiology. They are then held in place by the actions you do. This can be a great thing or a total disaster depending on the state and behaviours.

For example, if you are sitting with an upright posture, breathing slowly and deeply while focusing on how your body is improving you may feel motivated. As you are motivated you decide to exercise and eat healthily. This increases the chances you will keep an upright posture, breathe slowly and think about how your body is improving. The behaviour cycle fuels itself and keeps things on track.

The opposite version of this could be you are slumped in a chair with an irregular shallow breathing pattern. Your mind is focused on how you can never get in shape and the various problems you have in life. This combines to make you feel down and demotivated. As you are feeling this way you spend the evening on the sofa watching TV and eating junk. This results in you spending yet more time slumped over, breathing irregularly and focusing on your negative thoughts. The cycle fuels itself further keeping you stuck and despondent.

In health & fitness terms there are certain states that can help or hinder getting results. This could be how you feel while eating, when exercising or around your overall motivation. It is important to learn how to transition into the required states when they are needed.

Accessing your different states can be affected by your environment, the people around you and the specific area of your life. For example, it is common to see someone very motivated around others in say their work place but drop into a predominantly demotivated state with their health and fitness when at home alone. This is fairly common and it can be changed over time.

Your goal is to develop enough of the necessary motivational states to be active when you need them and also learn how to break out of destructive states. Common ones to work on include being relaxed when eating, having fun while exercising and breaking out of a binge eating episode or a prolonged period of being stuck in the house and not moving. This would also include your ability to edge your way out of more general low motivation periods.

*****

Each of these different sources of motivation may play a role in your success. For quickest improvements in your motivation you should address the area you need the most. However, it is often hard to specifically work out your needs so it is usually wise to apply all of the techniques at some point during your transformation. This will really lay the foundations for ongoing motivation. When you are more motivated you will be able to put more effort into the other areas within the transformation cycle.

Plans & Actions

The more motivation you consistently experience the more energy you will have to put into your efforts. This can be directed into the many different types of plans within the transformation cycle which include;

<u>A Unified Transformation Plan</u>

Traditionally, your 'plan' would just mean your nutrition and exercise routine. A Unified plan covers everything that you do. This includes all protocols, behaviours, experiments or plans that you follow. It is your roadmap for success.

A unified plan is designed to make use of everything you are learning about in this book and within the Grand Unified Theory. It can be very simple by covering just one or two areas or more extensive. The target is to help you achieve your goals and be able to maintain the results thereafter. Once designed an effective unified plan is never set in stone or is too rigid. It is adapted based on how you respond to it.

For optimal results you will want to use a unified plan that covers as many areas as possible from within the transformation cycle. There are example plans in section 4. Within the unified plan there are different types of protocols / plans that are used. These include:

Body Re-Composition Plans

This refers to the more traditional nutrition and exercise schemes. They provide the framework of what you should be doing within your food and movement. These can be formal, such as calorie based diets, meal plans or exercise routines. Alternatively, they can be informal and use principles like eating more vegetables or doing some activity every day.

Though conventional diet and exercise plans may have a low long term success rate on their own they do have a powerful role to play in getting results. They can be used to deliver predicable results, develop specific skills and provide structure to your approach.

The key to optimising these types of strategies is that they must have a high focus on sustainability and adherence. This involves allowing for taste, convenience, socialising and personal preferences.

Behaviour Change & Influencing Plans

The focus with these methods is to change the way you act or alter the likelihood of taking action in a future scenario. They include the protocols used to develop your motivation, neural connections, stress management and more. They also cover special methods that could be necessary in areas such as improving body image, binge eating or food addiction. These plans look nothing like any of the usual ones associated with food or movement. They may involve doing meditations, reading a book on a particular subject or changing just one of your behaviours for three days to train your brain.

You can do these protocols alongside the body re-composition plans though sometimes methodologies in this area may force you to pause or change your nutrition or exercise routine.

Long Term Maintenance Plan

When you have achieved your goal there would be some sort of a long term plan in place to ensure you are able to resist the negative influences and general erosion of healthy behaviours that happen over time.

It is pretty easy to maintain results and much easier than changing your body the first time round. The plan uses different areas from the transformation cycle to maintain current behaviour patterns and habits. It is about ensuring every month or two you do a few key actions to stay on track.

Medical Based Plans

It can be the case that you need to follow protocols to address your health issues given to you by your Doctor, e.g. mental health issues such as medications for severe depression. These protocols are sometimes needed just to be able to function at a base level to follow the kind of plans presented in this book. Other areas may include if you have a severely compromised digestive system, hormonal issues as well as numerous other possible health conditions.

Specificity of Plans

All plans would be tailored to the appropriate level of the person following it. This is related to the class of body shape and current behaviours. If you are eating a few chocolate bars a day you probably do not need to be worrying about the best way to cook vegetables. Likewise, if you have always struggled with exercise then you need to focus on changing your behaviours around fitness rather than trying to follow a training routine used by top athletes.

Variety of Plans

Too often we become fixated in our approach to get in shape and try to use one plan for life. It is very common for people to get great results using a method for a couple of months. At this point they should change to another strategy or develop a different skill but most become too rigid in their approach. Best results come from using a variety of methods / plans.

Actions

This area of the transformation cycle specifically mentions both plans and actions as they are not the same. A plan is your proposed tasks to do while your actions are what you actually end up doing. All too often what someone says they follow will in no way resemble what they actually do. Actions create results so it is important to judge your plan on what you actually did.

Another element to taking action is that you do not have to use a formal plan to be able to get results. Some of the previous transformation stories showed how results were possible by just changing one or two elements. Adding in 10 minutes of daily journaling, spending more time with a fit friend, eating out of smaller plates or taking a break from fat loss every few weeks could be enough to change your results. This hardly sounds like the most extravagant overhaul but key actions from within the transformation cycle areas can produce spectacular results.

Fat Loss Skills - The Four Phases

Whatever elements you do or do not do within your unified plan much of your success is going to come back to how well you have developed your fat loss skills. It is a misconception that changing body shape is just about being able to lose fat. This is just the first of the four skills you need. These are;

Losing fat – This is basis of any transformation, when you commit to it, do you know what to do and are you able to actually stick to the plan to lose fat? As discussed previously the simpler and less extreme your plan the easier it will be to follow. Likewise, the quicker the speed of fat loss or the longer you try to follow the plan then the harder it becomes.

It is a skill to be able to stick to your plan and balance the delicate temptations of wanting to get results vs wanting to eat more food or laze around watching TV. It is an ongoing self-negotiation. The better you are at dealing with yourself the better you will become at losing fat. Despite this almost everyone has lost body fat before, even if just for short periods of time. Most people are better at losing fat than they would think but they struggle with the other three skills.

Returning To Breakeven – After going through a period of losing weight at some point you will need to stop either because you are at your goal or you need a break. It is this transition from fat loss to break even that many people struggle with. It could be that you can lose fat without a problem but the moment you finish you seem to eat badly for the same amount of time you ate well. This means you eventually end up back at square one.

If this pattern happens to you it simply means you have not developed the skill of returning to normal eating after a period of weight loss. Through practice you will be able to recognize how to increase food in a measured way and drop into maintenance. This will allow you to sustain your new lower body fat levels. Doing this takes practice and it is not a knowledge issue.

Being able to eat at breakeven thresholds is also ideal for gaining muscle as it allows you to optimise growth while not gaining fat. The maintenance intake level should also be your target if you are looking to develop your health. If you eat at this threshold with the right healthy foods for your body it will boost your health and metabolism.

Restarting Fat Loss – As you will probably need to take a few breaks between fat loss periods to get to your ultimate goal you will need to develop your ability to restart the fat loss process. If you can add this skill of being able to lose weight again after a break even period at maintenance you will fairly effortlessly be able to use on / off periods. This is the most effective strategy for long term fat loss.

It is again a skill to be able to edge yourself from breakeven into another period of being in a calorie deficit. It is about managing your imagery of perceived difficulty and enjoyment of the tasks. It is about starting in some small way which creates more energy as a result. It is almost like a tiny version of the stages of change outlined previously at the start of the transformation cycle.

Returning to Break Even during an Overeating Period – Another element you probably need is the skill to snap out of a period of overeating and get back to break even. This could be after a week's holiday, a crazy weekend or two months of work stress. The faster you can get away from overeating and back to breakeven the quicker you will minimise the damage.

If you can avoid back tracking with your weight it can be a game changer. Many people expend a lot of time and energy every year simply removing the few Kg they have just gained. If you could find a way to break even then those same losses would edge you closer and closer to the final goal.

A common problem here is your desire to jump immediately from an overeating period into a fat loss phase. All too often when overeating, your attempt to go straight into fat loss will extend your overeating period. The ability to return to break even is adequate enough and then in due course you could worry about returning to a fat loss phase if applicable.

*****

These methods are developed by purposefully planning periods where you lose fat vs break even. This on-off approach will train these skills. It is very beneficial to be able to move in and out of fat loss. It can allow people with special considerations to get results, e.g. if you have binge eating tendencies, strong menstrual pains etc. In these scenarios you can decide when and for how long to try to lose fat and ensure it corresponds to when you are feeling your best. You would then break even during the more the difficult times and repeat this pattern for a far more enjoyable and easier path to your end goal.

As you develop these skills you will become more and more successful at changing your body and being able to maintain the results.

Neural Connections

Your neural pathways are what govern your habits and the vast majority of your behaviour patterns. While motivation and willpower capture most of the headlines it often gets forgotten why you even need motivation in the first place. The reason most people search for motivation is to get them to do the things they are not doing naturally. Your neural connections are those natural behaviour patterns.

If you were to develop a set of neural pathways that automatically made you eat healthy foods in moderate amounts while exercising regularly you would not need much motivation at all.

When your connections support the behaviours that bring results you will find health & fitness goals become not just attainable but much easier than you would ever have thought. For example, if you have never smoked in your life, how much willpower does it take for you to not smoke? Compare that to someone who is trying to quit. The reason willpower is important is that you need it to retrain your neural systems. Once they are retrained life is much easier.

You can create neural pathways to do something new, e.g. train yourself to like exercise, or you can collapse neural circuits to stop your bad behaviours e.g. train yourself to not to eat so much junk food.

Habits are the end product of neural connective training and will determines how you act the majority of the time. Your neural connections will also determine the feelings you will experience in any given situation. This will determine how you will act in non-regular situations that come up in life.

If you are looking for reasons why you have failed to get the results you want so far then this area may provide you with the answers you are looking for.

In most transformation stories you can normally see all sorts of ways the person has changed their neural programming. For example, in a blog about cyclists[33] who each lost over 45kg you could see that they didn't just follow an exercise plan using a bike but they fell in love with the sport of cycling. This could only happen by completely retraining the neural connections around cycling and exercise.

Despite the power of working on this area it is very rare for anyone to actively engage on a programme to develop connections even though it is quite simple to do. This is because very few people in the health & fitness focus on creating habits.

"Good" & "Bad" Neural Pathways

The actual neural pathways are inanimate. They are just operating away within your mind and body. In this sense they are neutral, however, we often label the behaviours they produce as "Good" or "Bad".

The best way to view any behaviour from a neural point of view is to compare it against its counter behaviour and see it as two sides competing against each other. For example, 'I eat too much chocolate' or 'I drink too much wine when out' should be viewed alongside an alternative option such as 'I eat healthy snacks' or 'I enjoy a night out without drinking'.

At this point you can then weigh up how many connections you have in support of the "bad" behaviour e.g. eating chocolate, drinking alcohol, and compare it to the amount of connections you hold in favour of the "Good" behaviours, e.g. eating healthy snacks, socialising without alcohol etc.

The relative balance between these two sides will predict which behaviour gets done most frequently. The diagram below shows this situation;

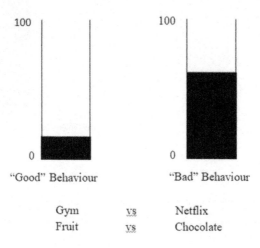

In the above example you would expect the "bad" behaviours of Netflix and eating chocolate to fairly regularly win the battle of the two behaviours. This is due to the large amount of connections to these "bad" behaviours and much less to the "good" ones. If you really wanted to go to the gym or eat fruit you would need to use your motivation and willpower to override your inclined desires for the Netflix or chocolate.

When you look at every behaviour / neural pathway with this competing model between the "good" and "bad" behaviours you will find six main possible outcomes, these are;

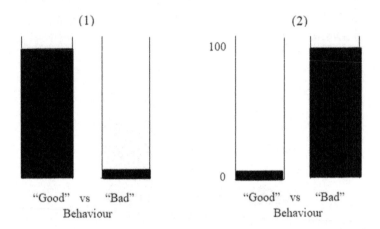

(1) In this scenario you will mostly do the good behaviours as there are a large amount of connections to doing them and almost zero connections to the opposite bad behaviours. This could be having some fruit for breakfast vs having a chocolate bar at 7am. Maybe it is going for a Sunday afternoon walk vs going to the pub. It would require almost no motivation to choose the fruit or walk rather than the chocolate or pub if these were your connections.

(2) In this example you will end up doing the bad behaviour as there are a large number of connections to them and pretty much no connections to the opposing good behaviour. This could be eating junk relaxing in front of the TV on a Saturday night compared to the idea of doing a healthy weekend juice 'detox'. To choose the detox it would take a huge amount of willpower as you would need to resist your cravings and desires to eat and drink. Even if you did do it you would probably feel pretty miserable during it.

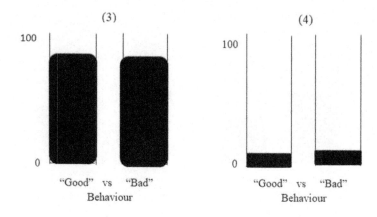

(3)

(4)

"Good" vs "Bad"
Behaviour

"Good" vs "Bad"
Behaviour

(3) In this situation you will find yourself jumping from the good to the bad behaviours and vice versa. The strong connections to both means you are ready to do either depending on the circumstances. You could be in the gym every day for a month or at home watching Netflix for three weeks. Which behaviour gets done is not an issue of willpower per se but more about other influences and triggers, e.g. maybe when your partner is home you always watch TV but if they are out at work you go to the gym.

(4) In this case you will not take much action in either of these behaviours. There are very few connections to doing the good behaviour or the bad one. As a person you would have little interest in this whole area, e.g. you have no interest in fasting yet also do not like overeating, or maybe you have never done formal exercise but you are generally active. To get yourself to do the good behaviour you would need to use motivation to take action and/or or understand the reasons for doing it.

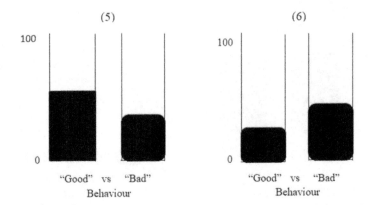

(5) In this scenario you will do the good behaviour a lot of the time but you still have enough bad connections to do both of the behaviours regularly within your natural patterns, e.g. you mostly eat healthy lunches but a couple of times a week you get a unhealthy take out. If you wanted to completely eliminate the bad behaviour you would need to use some of your willpower.

(6) The final scenario would see your bad behaviour winning the majority of the times but there are still enough good connections to have both behaviours regularly within your behaviour patterns, e.g. you try to eat a healthy dinner but generally eat too many pizzas and burgers. To ensure you do more of the good behaviours than the bad you will need some motivation and willpower to disrupt your current balance.

Your Connection Patterns

The ideal situation would be to have many connections to all of the needed good behaviours and very few to the bad ones (scenario 1 above). However, you may find you are starting out with the exact opposite, you have very few connections to the good behaviours and plenty towards the bad (scenario 2).

To rebalance your connections you have two options, you can look to build up the neural connections to the good behaviours or reduce the connections to the bad behaviours.

These do not have to be done simultaneously. For example, instead of trying to give up junk food you could instead focus on finding ways to enjoy eating enough protein, vegetables and healthy foods during the day. Over time this would build up your connections towards healthy eating even though you have not stopped your junk food. This would create the situation in scenario (6) above and then scenario (3). At that point you could look to reduce the connections you have to the bad behaviour to eventually end up in scenario (1).

Accept Your Connections

Connections are formed by repeating an action over and over again. To this point, any bad behaviour you have right now or the lack of good behaviour is simply because of the number of times you have repeated it. You do not need to judge, hate or look down upon your bad behaviours. There is nothing wrong with you. If you do not like exercise or lower calorie foods relax! You can develop any attribute you so desire over time.

Forming New Neural Connections

The process to create new neural connections is as follows –

*****

-Do a form of the desired behaviour (Easiest version to do).
-Celebrate and feel good about doing the task.
-Repeat the task soon and regularly (Increase task difficulty).
-Celebrate doing the task once more.
-Repeat the process.

*****

Neural connections are created through repeated actions. The time it takes to form a neural pathway is a combination of repetitions done vs emotions experienced upon doing it. The less emotion involved the more reps needed and vice versa. For this reason it is really important to celebrate and feel good about any efforts you take when trying to form a new connection.

When it comes to repeated actions it is the number of times you do a behaviour that is more important than how you actually do it, e.g. if developing your desire to exercise then each time you start a session you develop your exercise neural connections, it is not relevant whether you do 5 or 50 minutes exercising after you have started. Therefore, behaviour wise it would be better to do seven 5 minute runs in a week than one 50 minute jog.

When you focus on increasing how many times you do an action rather than how well you do the behaviour it helps with adherence. It is much easier to be consistent with a shorter and easier option.

Very often you are unable to do the full task through a lack of knowledge or because it is too intimidating. In this case start off with the easiest version of the task that you are ok with doing. For example, if the gym is too intimidating then maybe start with walking and a home exercise video. When ready to try the gym, maybe you get a friend to take you when it is quiet. Over time you will become confident enough to use the gym on your own even when it is busy.

In general, forming connections is slower than breaking them down. One instance where it can appear to be much faster is if you used to do the behaviour previously. If you played tennis as a kid it would be quicker for you to awaken the old connections than for someone else to form new ones for the first time.

While it is not complicated to create a new connection it does take many repetitions to build it into the mental circuitry. The best way to accelerate the process is through using high levels of emotion if possible while doing the tasks.

Maintaining Connections

Connections are fairly fluid in that they increase and decrease in excitation based on how many times they are performed and the emotion experienced alongside them. One of the better ways to imagine them is that they are like a path through a forest.

To initially create a path it takes a fair bit of work to cut down and flatten the vegetation. Once formed the path is maintained through it being used regularly. If the path is not used for a while it slowly begins to become more overgrown. This makes it a little harder to move through it and if this lack of use continues over a longer period then the pathway becomes blocked.

At this point, if you wanted to use it again, you would need to cut it down and flatten the vegetation once more. Even though this would take effort it would be easier to cut down the old path than it would be to form a new route for the first time.

Neural pathways are exactly the same, they take effort to create the circuit for the first time but once formed can be kept open by using them regularly. If you fail to use them then they will become less responsive. If unused for a long period it would feel like you have never done that behaviour. However, it will be easier to get back into it in the future if you were to start doing it again. This works for both good and bad behaviours.

As mentioned if you loved a certain sport or exercise when young it will not take that many repetitions to rekindle your love for it now. However, it is also common for smokers to quit for many years and then go back to smoking during a stressful period. The same neural connections process can work in your favour or against you.

For most people they simply need to be aware that their connections need a little attention occasionally to ensure the neural pathways are maintained going forwards into the future. This is the basis of the methods used in a long term maintenance plan.

Breaking Neural Connections –

The point of rewiring your connections to food and exercise is not to make you into a Saint who never eats badly or is so obsessed with exercise they have no time for anything else. The goal is to give you choice and freedom.

Choice means it is as easy to say yes as it is to say no in any circumstance, this means sometimes you will do the 'bad' behaviour while other times you will not. It is easy to behave with moderation when you are comfortable with saying no. This is important because almost everyone can achieve their goals using moderation. It is fine to sometimes do the "bad" behaviour if other times you will choose the "good" option.

When it comes to breaking neural connections you will usually need a little willpower and to feel motivated. Most forms of breaking a connection comes through structured abstinence exercises.

The way your brain works is that you get a cue/trigger e.g. you finish work, walk into the supermarket or get home. This causes the brain to have a neural spike (brain waves increase, biochemical changes). At this point you feel an urge to act in response to this sensation, e.g. grab some food, pour a glass of wine etc.

To break this cycle you will need to sit through the trigger (stimulation of brain waves) and then wait until you are past the point of the response behaviour. This is the basis of breaking a neural connection. You would then need to repeat it again, this next time the neural signal will be a tiny bit weaker, again you must sit through the signal until past the point of the response behaviour.

This process can be continued to greatly reduce and completely transform the way you act around your triggers. Eventually this will break down the neural connections to your bad behaviours.

You may be surprised by how quickly the connection can be changed and reduced. For most behaviours it takes somewhere between 3 to 10 attempts to collapse the vast majority of the connections. For example, say you eat two chocolate cookies at 3pm every day. To reduce this connection you would simply need to not eat anything around 3pm for between 3- 10 days. At this point the brain would no longer behave in the same way to the 3pm cue.

Variety of Stimuli

An important element to this process is ensuring you have addressed the various similar stimuli that each connection to a bad behaviour may hold. For example, if you have a glass of wine, it is likely you will experience it differently on a Tuesday compared to a Saturday night. This is because Saturday usually has associations to not working, socialising, relaxing and so forth which Tuesday does not. Therefore it would be harder for most people to not drink on a Saturday.

To break your connections you will need to ensure you have addressed the various different stimuli. In general it is advised to start with the easiest connection to sit through then build from there, e.g. focus on having a healthy work lunch on a Monday over Friday when it is Take out Friday at work.

It is the lack of confronting the various elements that trips most people up. This is shown every year when many people partake in dry January where they give up alcohol for the month. This is a great gesture however most people decide to spend the whole month inside and never go out to socialise.

The result is they have not addressed the full spectrum of their neural cues around drinking. This means they are no better at not drinking in social situations after a month off alcohol than they were before. It would be far more prudent to go out during dry January while still not drinking. If you did this it would have long lasting benefits for the rest of the year.

The same happens when you are motivated and on a healthy diet. Do not drop your social life and avoid going out. You will miss out on a huge opportunity to change your connections. If you went to your usual environments but behaved in a different way you will create long term changes that would continue to give you results way after you run have out of motivation on this current effort.

Celebration of Success

An important element to retraining the brain is celebrating success. Emotion is one of the fastest ways to imprint a neural circuit. A very painful or joyous event will create immediate neural pathways. Therefore you need to be open to feeling good when you make positive strides with your behaviours.

As discussed previously with the rules of progress you need to take the attitude that if you do any effort to change your behaviours you should celebrate what you have done. This taps into the dopamine pathways to feel good. Avoid the temptation to focus on how you were not perfect, how much more you could have done or what someone else would do. All this takes away the positive feelings that will help re-programme your brain.

Many people avoid celebrating success as they feel failure is around the next corner and they will soon mess up again as has happened in the past. While this cautious feeling is understandable it slows behaviour change. Each successful repetition of a specific behaviour tips the balance slightly towards better neural programming. Therefore it is important to simply celebrate this success in that moment, forget what the future may bring and enjoy your victory that day.

Rewiring the Craving

A powerful way to change a bad behaviour is to rewire the feeling associated with the cue/stimuli. If you can change a positive feeling around a trigger into a negative feeling or repulsion you will transform your behaviour pattern immediately. You would have seen this happen if you have ever got horribly drunk and ill from a specific drink, you will often never be able to drink it again due to your association to that negative experience.

To rewire a craving you need to feel a genuine negative emotion (as in the drink example above) or experience new thought about what that behaviour means. For example, eating a bar of chocolate for most is a pleasurable activity. However, for some, eating a chocolate bar is symbolic of a bad period in their life and living in a way they never want to repeat again. When the thought of eating chocolate represents something much greater than the action itself you will change how you feel and act.

To create such a transition in belief you will need to spend time considering the consequences of certain actions and look at how they have affected your life up until now and moving forwards into the future.

Dopamine System

Another aspect to your neural programming is your relationship to dopamine, which we discussed around your rules of progress. Dopamine gives you immediate rewards of feeling good. It is designed to help you choose good behaviours and reward you for being on the right track for achieving a goal.

However, dopamine is stimulated by various other things such as high calorie foods, social interaction, anything sexually related (porn), receiving rewards, drugs and much more. These artificial dopamine stimulators can completely disrupt the natural balance of this system.

The reason your phone and social media are so addictive is that it provides so many ways to trigger dopamine. It could be you receive a new message, see a funny photo, chat to someone new and much more. In addition to this you do not know what you are going to get so the excitement and anticipation of reward stimulates yet more dopamine.

In health & fitness terms if you have associated food as the primary way for achieving dopamine stimulation it will be hard to simply stop eating. Genuine food addiction is dopamine based in the same way as other addictions such as gambling, drinking, drugs etc. However, it can be hard to identify food addiction as many other factors also influence eating as well.

Addressing your behaviours via an angle of dopamine is about changing your foods, handling the anticipation of eating and looking at your dopamine related activities. In some cases you will need to allow this system to rebalance itself by temporarily reducing all sources of dopamine stimulation.

Emotions & Stress

One of the biggest influences in regards to causing you to fail will be stress. It is very common that you know what to do but the moment stress appears you end up not doing it.

Stress is the collection of negative thoughts and emotions that you are experiencing. Finding and implementing ways to reduce and manage your stress is a powerful weight loss strategy. When stressed you will usually eat too much food and become inconsistent with your exercise and movement. If you happened to react to stress by eating vegetables and exercising a lot then this would not be an area of concern during a body transformation but that rarely happens.

There are different ways you may act when stressed, you may end up eating a lot of the same "bad" foods, e.g. the whole tub of ice cream, or maybe you stop moving and spend the whole weekend watching Netflix. Alternatively, the effect of stress can be quite subtle in that it may simply cause you to make many small errors within your health and fitness behaviours, e.g. grabbing an unnecessary snack on the way home or eating slightly larger portions. These actions can stop progress even though you are still mostly doing your plan.

How well you handle stress comes back to what stress management techniques you do or do not use and how much stress is within your life. There are two main types of stress management technique; coping behaviours and reduction techniques. In addition to this you can investigate the causes of stress to lower your overall levels.

It is not necessary to have a stress free life or to resolve all of your problems/issues to get results. You just need to change your response so you keep moving and do not overeat to any great extent during a stressful period.

Not all bad eating is because of stress. It could be your neural programming is at the heart of the problem due to the connections you have to "bad" foods. Maybe you are following a food plan too low in protein, taste or overall calories which are causing your food cravings and binges. For this reason it is important to look at emotional eating while addressing other areas within the transformation cycle to cover all the bases.

Definitions & Types of Stress

'Stress' comes from different sources, some of which are more obvious than others. The main stress sources are:

A Racing Mind – Too Many Thoughts per Minute

When your mind is racing with too many thoughts per minute, be it numerous different thoughts or the same few ones repeating over and over again you will feel stressed. The thoughts do not necessarily need to be negative though they generally will be. In this situation it is important to slow the mind down. This type of stress is helped greatly by moving the body and meditation methods.

Surface Level Negative Emotions

This is the typical stress generated by your emotions in response to what is happening in life. It could be you feel worried, angry, sad, guilty or a mixture of these and much more. All sorts of day to day events cause us stress including arguments, work projects, children, relationships, family gathering, the news, friendships and so forth.

The surface level refers to the permanence of the emotional events. We encounter many events in day to day life that can stress us out but the moment they have passed the stress usually goes away with it. The best way to handle this type of stress is to use a technique to counter or reduce the emotions and then if possible take action to resolve the cause of it.

It may be that you also need you to examine some of your own personal beliefs that could be causing more stress than is necessary within these situations. This can include your personal expectations, perfectionism and your actions.

Underlying Negative Emotions

A large source of stress comes from your thoughts about your past, present and future. They not only affect your emotional health but they can also influence how you react to everyday events therefore causing more surface level stresses.

Your past may have various unresolved emotions from events that have happened when you were young or more recently. This may range from small to large emotional events and includes traumatic memories. Your current evaluations of life refer to your expectations of what you should have achieved or who you should be vs how you actually perceive yourself. This can result in feelings of shame, guilt, sadness or failure. Future concerns can range from small worries to larger fears about your future including the issues of life and death.

Physical Pain

When you are in physical pain it can be a significant stress that leads to disruptions in your physiology and psychological well-being. It also frequently results in emotional eating. Sources of pain include injuries sustained previously, health conditions, on-going joint problems or illness.

Total Stress

The above stressors combine to give a "total amount of stress" that you are experiencing at any one time. I call this your emotional terrain. There can be a large difference in the amount of stress in your life compared to someone else due to your current circumstances and the experiences you have been through.

There are also individual differences in how you experience stress with some people more susceptible to it than others due to our biology or the mood state they are in, e.g. how many people's problems disappear in life the moment they fall in love? Stress will also vary greatly within your own life at different times based on the circumstances at that moment. This can be summed up in the diagram below;

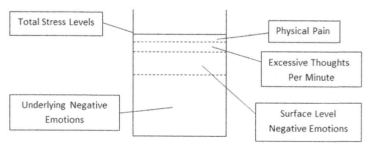

Coping With Stress –

The way a certain amount of stress affects your health & fitness comes back to your coping mechanisms. Your ability to handle stress can be done via positive coping methods, e.g. exercise, hobbies, meditation or in ways with more negative consequences e.g. eating junk food, drinking, watching TV etc. The greater your ability to handle stress without relying on negative strategies the better it is for you, your life and your health and fitness.

Total Stress vs Types of Stress vs Coping Abilities

When we consider the different sources of stress and your ability to cope with it then a few different scenarios could occur. These are outlined below –

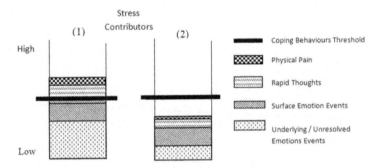

In the above scenarios (1) and (2) we can see that both people have the same coping threshold but in scenario (2) they are experiencing much less stress in their life than the other. This may be because they have a less stressful life, are naturally less susceptible to experiencing stress or perhaps they use methods to reduce their stress levels.

In practical terms you would expect the person in scenario (2) to be able to follow their health & fitness plans much easier than (1) if all else is equal. To improve the chances of getting results in scenario (1) you would look to use techniques to reduce stress or improve coping strategies.

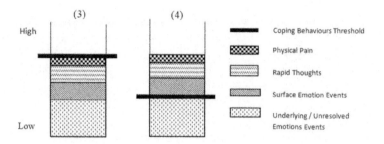

In scenarios (3) and (4) the people are experiencing the same levels of stress yet (3) has a much greater coping abilities. This means they can handle their current stress levels without resorting to negative behaviours such as excess eating or drinking. It is therefore fairly likely they will be able to get results going forwards.

For the person in scenario (4) their lesser coping abilities mean they are unable to handle the stress they are under. Therefore, you would expect their food or exercise routine to deteriorate due to it and they will struggle to get results. Going forwards, person (4) should look to develop his stress coping abilities to get better results. They would also benefit by reducing their stress levels.

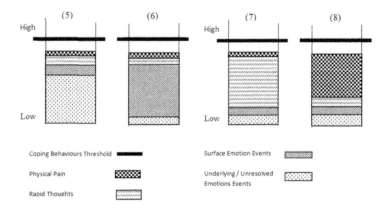

In scenarios (5), (6), (7) and (8) they all have the same levels of stress and coping ability, therefore an equal likelihood of achieving their health and fitness goals. However, you can see the source of the stress is different between the scenarios.

In scenario (5) it is underlying emotional events from the past that dominate the causes of stress, e.g. they had an abusive childhood. In (6) it is current day to day events and stresses e.g. their child is ill and they have a big work presentation. For scenario (7) the person is just experiencing too many rapid thoughts, e.g. trying to decide between two jobs offers and plan their wedding. In the final scenario (8) actual physical pain is the major cause of stress in the person's life, e.g. they have a broken collar bone and a horrible cold.

The four scenarios would need to use different methods to reduce the stress. While meditating would really help the racing mind in (7) it would probably not be so beneficial for dealing with an abusive childhood (5) or physical pain (8).

There is no set pattern to knowing which stress cause affects you the most. For some people, maybe one source predominates while others are more balanced between the four.

There are also no hard set rules for any of these issues, for example, having an abusive childhood doesn't necessarily mean you have traumatic memories and likewise being in physical pain may not represent a stress to you. The point to note is that based on the major stressor you experience, the best therapeutic intervention / method to help you will vary. For this reason you would want to develop a broad set of tools to handle what stresses life throws at you.

General 'Stress' Vs Crisis Response

When very stressful events happen (a crisis) there is usually a spike in the stress response. This will engage your fight or flight system and you may even enter a state of shock. This happens in times of bereavement, if you lose your job, ending of relationships, traumatic incidents and so forth.

During this period most people find they often do not eat that much food due to being in full on crisis management mode. However, as the dust settles your nervous system calms and the above emotional levels vs coping mechanisms balance begins to display itself again. In some circumstances, a crisis can leave you with trauma / PTSD type conditions. This not only affects underlying emotions but can also shut down the goal focused parts of your brain. This means you will appear demotivated and this can affect all areas of your life.

Changing Your Body vs Resolving Life's Problems

The goal of addressing your stress is to ensure it is under enough control to not ruin your ability to stick to your plan. It is not about solving every problem you may have in life. Instead, you are trying to disconnect your feelings of stress from overeating or being sedentary. This is done by either changing your reactions to the stress itself or experiencing less of it.

Avoid making your stress levels or negative emotions an excuse about why you cannot achieve your goals. You do not need 10 years of therapy to change your body shape. You do not need to solve every issue you may have and you can still get into amazing shape even if the rest of your life is a 'mess'.

All you need to do is nudge your stress levels a little downwards and/or adjust how you react to it so it does not affect your health and fitness behaviours.

Handling Stress

To counter the influence of stress there are different options available to you. These include;

Stress Coping Approaches – There is a wide selection of behaviours that allow you to cope with stress. The big three around stress management are eating healthy foods, daily movement and getting adequate sleep. These carry the biggest impact on how you handle stress. In addition to these there are various other techniques that you may find beneficial. The stronger your stress coping behaviours the more stress you can handle without eating junk or drinking.

Stress / Emotional Reduction Strategies – These methods directly lower the amount of stress and emotion you are experiencing. While stress coping behaviours allow you to handle more stress, these techniques look to reduce your actual stress levels. There are many methods you can use, some of these can be done on your own while others involve coaches or group work.

It is important to have access to techniques you can do alone so you are able to reduce stress whenever you need to. Solo techniques can include meditation, journaling and various stress therapies such as Emotional Freedom Technique (EFT).

Most people make their best strides when part of structured groups or if working directly with a trained professional. A combination of expertise, commitment and an environment focused on change will allow for personal growth around stress. There are a host of techniques and methodologies that can help reduce it under these circumstances such as therapy, counselling, eye movement therapies and much more.

Resolving The Causes of Stress – Long term stress management should also look to address some of the underlying causes of it. While stress will always be present in your life to some degree you can reduce the amount experienced through a variety of methods. Some of these look at what you need to improve in your life to cut off stress at its source while others look at how you perceive stress, both the framework you use to evaluate it and the meaning assigned to it.

*Note - If you suffer from physical pain you should also look into the various pain management techniques. They are beyond the scope of this book.

*****

When you start using methods to counter stress it will often be the difference between you winning and losing in a 50/50 situation, e.g. you are tempted to order a take out, you walk past some nice smelling street food, you are not sure if feeling up for the exercise class. A less stressed you may well pick the better option in all of these situations. A few victories per week can be the difference between great results or none at all. The more methods you are familiar with and the greater your skills in using them the better your ability to handle stress will become.

Fitness Personality

Your Fitness Personality represents who you are as a person within the confines of health & fitness. It considers how you identify yourself, the self-talk that you use, which groups you consider yourself a part of and the environment you have created in your life. It is the difference between following a plan and doing something because that is who you are. It is also a way to predict your future results.

Your fitness personality includes your class of body shape, which is your outward projection to the world and your Fitness identity, which is your internal representation.

The Seven Classes of Body Shape

We have already touched upon the different classes. You have seen how they represent the time, effort, skill and focus needed to produce a certain body type. They are not better or worse than each other but just reflect how much input is needed to achieve them and therefore the type of advice you should be given.

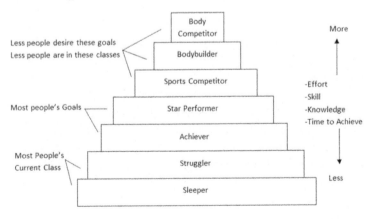

At a basic outward physical level the classes are separated by;

Body Fat – The body fat levels generally go down as you move up the pyramid of classes. The bodybuilder categories will often use bulking and cutting periods so that they have phases every year when they are very low in body fat yet are at higher levels outside of these periods.

Muscle Mass – The amount of muscle you have separates the higher body type classes on the pyramid with increasing amounts of muscle needed for each class further up.

*****

Outside of the physical external traits there are various behaviour traits that can differentiate between the body shape classes. In general, the higher up the pyramid you go the 'better' the behaviours in each trait need to be. The main traits include;

Exercise Frequency – How many times you exercise per week and also how consistent you are throughout the year.

Exercise Knowledge – How much you know about exercise, both how to do it and why. Certain body type classes need a much greater knowledge around exercise.

Exercise Enjoyment – How much you enjoy exercise and integrate it within your life as a fun thing to do.

Nutrition Knowledge – What you know and understand about nutrition in both a theory sense and also at an individual level tailored for your body.

Nutrition Consistency – How good you are with your nutrition both across a week and also throughout the year.

Eating Out – The amount of times you order a takeaway to eat at home as well as how often you go to restaurants.

Alcohol – How much you drink and the pattern of your drinking behaviour which may include binge drinking.

Fitness – This varies between the classes and is based on your exercise skills, consistency and individual goals.

Importance in Life – The significance you place on both the importance of body shape within your life and the role of your behaviours within your identity.

Daily Focus & Check In – This relates to how much you think about your goal and your body. It also includes how often you look in the mirror and check in on this goal area.

Social Ties – The way your fitness related behaviours integrate into your social life determines some of your results. People in certain classes have most of their social ties coming from their fitness. The bodybuilding classes usually have their focus on fitness take over their whole social life.

Stress Connection – How stress affects your eating patterns and exercise adherence is an important part of achieving year round consistency. This greatly influences results.

Use of Experts – The likelihood of using a professional or seeking the advice of an expert is inversely related to the external level of results, e.g. those in the best shape are most likely to use expert (despite probably needing it the least). While those who struggle with results are less likely to seek help (despite needing it the most).   An expert could be a sports coach, personal trainer, nutritionist or someone who has personally achieved a high level of results in specific area.

****

When you consider the above behaviours traits and beliefs alongside the external results you can form a clearer picture of the individual classes and what separates them.

Sleeper – With no real interest in this area their behaviours and results depend upon their natural behaviour patterns. Typically for most people in this class they have a low level of knowledge around both exercise and nutrition. This contributes to poor nutrition consistency throughout the year and few if any exercise sessions. They eat out or have takeaways regularly, they lead a sedentary life, drink frequently and have social ties based around food and drink.

Struggler – The behaviour patterns of a struggler can appear very similar to a sleeper, the main difference is the importance and awareness they have around their body and wanting to improve their situation. Generally they will have a low and/or incomplete knowledge around exercise and nutrition. This means they struggle to be consistent across a week or a year in one or both areas. Often strugglers are ok with exercise, movement or nutrition but not with all three at the same time. The majority of their social ties are based around food or drink and stress will usually completely destroy their efforts. They rarely make use of an expert to change their body.

Achiever – They have managed to attain success, so they will have a fair level of knowledge in nutrition, exercise or both. An aspect of this would have crept into their identity, e.g. friends think they are the healthy one, the runner etc. Some social connections will be around fitness while alcohol will be controlled to some degree. Stress will still cause many problems but they may use exercise to counter some of its effects. What separates them from the struggler is usually the increased knowledge and skill around exercise and nutrition. They will often use an expert at some point to develop this.

Star Performer – With a good level of results star performers have managed to learn about and enjoy exercise. This means their fitness is a jump above the previous classes and they will have more muscle and be leaner. Nutrition knowledge and adherence will also be more consistent too. Their body and behaviours are a fairly important part of their identity and they use health & fitness for a part of their social interactions. Alcohol intake will be modest or not really part of their life. Stress will affect things but usually will not totally destroy their efforts like with the previous classes. They have almost always used an expert at some point for a period of time.

Sports Competitor – This class of body types are very good at exercise with both consistency and skills in how they train. The result is they have more muscle than the previous classes. A big part of their social life revolves around fitness and their identity is quite significantly based in their body and/or sport. Their nutrition skills and consistency are good and they use exercise as a primary way to handle stress. Alcohol intake will be controlled or not really part of their life. They almost always have used an expert for guidance.

Bodybuilder – They have the same high exercise skills and consistency as a sports competitor but their focus is solely on developing their body shape. With these techniques they train almost every day and have a fairly rigid routine with food. This allows them to build extra muscle compared to previous classes. They base their social life heavily around fitness, often training with other people. They exercise as a primary way to handle stress and their identity is very heavily based on their goals and actions. They have used expert advice at some point and usually at various stages.

Most people in this class have considered using performance enhancing drugs though only percentage actually will use them. The use of steroids can make up for having below par exercise and nutrition knowledge or general consistency.

Body Competitor – At this class of body shape their life is totally focused around their body and pursuit of their goals. Whether amateur or professional (make money from doing it) their exercise and nutrition is of the highest consistency. Their whole social life is based around the gym, their friendships are mostly with similar minded people and they pretty much do not drink alcohol nor have many meals out.

Stress does not affect consistency though may alter intensity within some of their actions. They will usually have an expert, or team of people helping them prepare for competitions. They would have seriously considered using drugs to aid performance with a large percentage having used something at some point during their life.

Interplay of Factors vs Body Class Achieved

When it comes to the above traits they all have an input upon the class you can and will achieve. For example, if your knowledge and skills around food, eating, exercise and stress management are at an achiever standard then you will no doubt be an achiever class body shape.

In some cases a very high level of skill within one area can raise your overall body class above the level you would be expected to be, for example, if you are a struggler with exercise yet your food & eating are that of bodybuilder's knowledge & discipline it would no doubt lift you to an achiever level.

The opposite also occurs, if you have a sports competitor level of exercise adherence and knowledge yet no control over your eating it would maybe drop you down the pyramid to achiever or struggler level. In general, this latter example is often the way things pan out, you are very good in some areas but lacking ability in others. It is often your weakest element that sets your overall level of results.

The interplay of different automatic behaviours shows itself in the variety of body shapes in the sleeper class. Those in the sleeper class give little mental focus to health & fitness. Therefore their results are due to their own natural behaviour patterns. While this is bad for most people some do just fine. If you learnt sensible portion control and good eating habits when young and/or naturally like some sort of activity e.g. walking, you could be an achiever body class level of results without any mental focus at all.

Your Current Class and Goal

You should look to identify your current class and then see where your goal body shape lies. For most people their goal is one or two classes above their current class in the pyramid. The majority of the population want to be an achiever (around goal body weight) or a star performer (lean, athletic and fit). When you know your goal you can work out the general specific standard needed to be successful. Using the traits above you can work backwards to see what to do.

For example, if you want to be a star performer yet are currently a struggler, you can use the knowledge about what it takes to achieve it, e.g. they all exercise 1-3+ times a week. So if your current exercise regime is inconsistent you would need to investigate how you can become more regular with your fitness. Perhaps your knowledge is lacking, maybe you need more social connections within your exercise framework or you need to develop your neural connections towards fitness training.

A simple way to understand more about your goal requirements is to spend time with people who are already at that body shape class. This allows you to see, feel and learn about what it takes to achieve your goal.

<u>Appearing In the Wrong Class</u>

You may have a friend who does everything 'wrong' yet is in great shape. These 'Fake Thin people' exist for a few reasons. One is they just have a stronger metabolism or are less inclined to store fat. This is the luck of your genetics. Other times they do many of the traits to get results but you do not notice. For example, you may see them eating a cake at the café but do not see them eating nothing until dinner, or they get drunk Saturday night but are very good during the week.

The opposite is when someone has a large amount of muscle and their lifestyle is almost a perfect match of a sports competitor or bodybuilder but they are never lean so they do not fit into any category. The bodybuilder classes often use bulking and cutting phases, which means at some point during the year you will be at lower body fat levels. However, if you never manage to achieve a lean physique from a cutting phase at any point then you would not truly represent that class. This may be from choice or from not having the needed fat loss skills.

The Problem of Changing Classes

Most people spend extended periods of time within the same class, you may progress or regress a little but you pretty much stay within the same bracket. It is difficult to jump to the class above because it requires a significant change in behaviour or thinking, or both. Through taking a multi-faceted approach as outlined in the transformation cycle you stand the best chance to transition a new body class and achieve your goals.

If your ultimate goal is two or more classes away then you will need to be patient. First change your mind set and body to that of the next class up. Once cemented there you can then look to continue the process of changing body shape classes.

Fitness Identity

This is how you see yourself, it is the language you use, the labels you live by, your personal values, the groups you consider yourself a part of and the environment you create for yourself. It is all the elements of self-identity but in the context that applies to your health & fitness.

How You View Yourself

The summation of your beliefs, experiences and memories combine to determine how you view yourself today. It is an important aspect in behaviour change because your brain will endeavour to act in line with the kind of person you think you are, e.g. if you see yourself as a runner it increases your running consistency, if you feel you are a sensible eater it will improve your eating habits. You would therefore want to develop any important behaviour to be part of your personality and identity.

The question of how long it takes to integrate behaviours into your identity is an interesting issue. For example, does going for one run make you a runner? What if you ran three times a week for ten weeks? There are no right answers to this but the key is how you perceive yourself. Often identity does not update itself as you would like and despite exercising a few times a week for many years you may still view yourself as the lazy overweight kid. To get around this you would need to examine the criteria you use for determining your own traits and characteristics.

The reason this subject is important is that to change and then maintain a different class of body type you often have to shift who you are identity wise. There is a different feel and approach to following a plan to change who you are as a person verses just trying to lose some body fat or tone up.

Groups You Identify With

An element of personal identity is the groups you consider yourself a part of and member within. Your group identity and self-identity are very similar at a practical level. When you see yourself as part of a group you will endeavour to conform to some of the behaviour norms as a member.

Sometimes you can exclude yourself from a group which could stop you trying to achieve your goals, e.g. I could never be an athlete (member of the athletes group), I could never be thin (thin persons' group). If you truly feel you could never be a certain way you may never get started.

The desire to not be seen as a member of a group is also a powerful motivational tool, e.g. I would never be a 'couch potato', or one of those 'lazy parents'.

All group identity comes with a set of assumed beliefs about the traits needed to be in that group and the required behaviours of those in it. Just like with self-identity there are interesting questions about the criteria of becoming a member of any one group. How would you need to act and for how long to be considered a member?

It is common for your own identity to not update itself into new groups even if you are doing most of the actions of the group members, e.g. you run 3 times a week for and have done a marathon yet still don't see yourself as a runner.

Values

Your general life values merge into your health & fitness and it is important to consider their influence on what you are trying to achieve. We often feel that we should be aiming to be perfect with our nutrition or should give up alcohol or ice cream forever. The fundamental assumption here is that your health & fitness should be your number one priority in life. However, what is most important comes to you comes back to your values and there is no right or wrong in this area.

Food, drink and TV are integrated parts of our society, customs and traditions. It is important you ask yourself what you are trying to achieve within your behaviours and check they align with your life values. It is ok to want to eat bad foods, enjoy meals out, get drunk or spend the day watching Netflix. Avoid the temptation to feel you have to give these all up. This is a personal decision based on how you want to live life (your values).

At the same time you also have your health & fitness goals which can and should be achieved in a complimentary way to your values. All too often you will follow plans designed for people who aim to be perfect with their health & fitness. This will fail you long term. There are various ways to get results yet still respect your present values.

You really see this issue with the conventional approach which has someone on an intense plan that is working yet has no long term sustainability. There is nothing wrong with following that plan short term but you have to honour your other desires, beliefs and values at some point.

If you would like to have health & fitness as your number one priority in life then you will need to be patient and use many of the methods in this section such as being around other people who already have this view. However, only a few people truly want to be this way and it is much easier to get results as a compromise within your current values than to completely create a new set of them.

Rituals

This refers to a sequence of activities that serve to reinforce your actions and cement your identity. There are symbolic rituals and behaviour rituals.

Symbolic rituals refer to actions that act as a marker of achievement. Society has various symbolic rituals such as marriage ceremonies, exams, graduation etc. These events represent the attainment of an outcome and this can often result in a transition in identity, e.g. after marriage you become a husband / wife.

Within health and fitness these events could be running a marathon, doing your first full pull up or getting back into your old jeans after having a baby. You can use these achievements to facilitate adopting new traits into your personality. For example, when you run a marathon you are officially a runner and an active person in your own mind.

After doing an event you can put up a symbol/object to remind you of your success. This could be having your marathon medal on the cabinet or putting up a photo of you and your baby back in your old jeans. These rituals are periodic in that you are not doing them every week.

Behaviour rituals refer to regular actions that you do which act as a framework to keep your behaviours in place as well as reinforcing your identity. These rituals could be planning your food for the day, doing a stretch routine each morning or playing a sport every summer.

You would want to periodically do some symbolic ritual events to aid in the change or confirmation of your identity. You would also want to establish a strong set of behaviour rituals to lock your good behaviours in place and also reinforce your current beliefs, behaviours and identity.

Self-talk

Your self-talk is both a reflection of your beliefs, identity and who you are but also a mechanism by which you can influence change. This includes what you say to yourself and the underlying questions your subconscious keeps asking you.

Most people remain who they are through a series of mantras, a statement or slogan you frequently repeat. The continued repetition of these catch phrases influences you to act a certain way. This can be a good or a bad thing depending upon the behaviours you keep repeating. You would want to change your self-talk so that it is supporting your goals.

Changing your self-talk is one part changing your words but a big part changing who you are at the same time. You can rarely get results with affirmations if not backed up by action. This is because taking action and gathering new evidence is the primary way to alter your thinking patterns. You would also look to consider the beliefs that lie behind your words, where they came from and what you would need to do to change these.

In regards to using new language patterns it is important you have congruence with your words. A congruent statement is one that is both true and believable. Avoid using fanciful contradictions and super positive affirmations. For example, avoid going from 'I never have any discipline around food' to 'I always eat perfectly'. It does not work in the real world as you will remember the many times you have eaten badly. A better statement would be 'I sometimes have control around food and I am gradually improving'. This is more truthful and encourages you to find examples of good eating.

Alongside this new language you would be doing actions to generate further evidence for your new beliefs and language patterns, e.g. If you did a week of sensible eating your 'sometimes controlled around food' would now have more memories to support it.

Fitness Environment

Your personality in all areas of life is influenced by other people and the circumstances around you. Likewise, you influence others as well. It is important to create an environment that supports and embeds your desired health & fitness behaviours. This was also discussed in the motivation section under goal environment.

Your environment provides not just motivation but also confirms your identity. If you change your environment it will aid in facilitating your identity changes. This may include developing new social connections, making use of coaches, joining groups, using test data and much more. These methods mostly involve other people as this is the most effective way to be influenced positively. In most cases there is only so far you or anyone can go on your own and thus you will need to be around other people in some capacity during a transformation.

Personal Growth

Achieving your health & fitness goals assumes you will feel a certain way when you get there. However, it could be that your goal has more influences upon it than just what will come as a result of changing your body or behaviours. In such cases you may need to work on specific areas that will create the changes you desire.

Personal growth happens from undertaking a new approach in some form. This could be taking a course, deciding to resolve an argument, joining a support group, taking on a challenge, working on addictions, taking a risk etc. This area contributes to identity development as you will view yourself through a new lens each time you make progress in a personal growth exercise.

Change & Development of Your Fitness Identity

To develop and change your identity you need to use a variety of methods. The more you culture your environment to aid your transition the more effortless this process becomes. This can be accelerated through clarification of identity goals and then the use of language and rituals to cement the changes in place. Any personal growth tasks in other areas of your life will usually also be beneficial to changing your fitness identity.

Time & Patience

Identity change happens on a slow scale. It is takes time to change how you view yourself, adjust your language and build new rituals or a more supportive environment. It is not really an area you can rush due to the feedback loop of identity vs behaviour. This process can be helped when you clarify the line between certain self-identities or the criteria to be in a particular group. It can take many months to years for true identity change to happen so you will need to be patient.

Consequence of Identity Change

A true change of identity is not something to take lightly. There may be some upheaval if developing a 'new you' means you are losing an 'old you'. We are often tested in life when events happen to us that challenge the view we have of our own identity and who we think we are. Achieving your goals is a good thing but it is still a significant change.

Any big change in how you view yourself affects your perceived place in the world. It has implications for life moving forward and consequences for decisions made in the past. This can all take a little mental processing and can involve some of the features seen in the process of loss akin to when you go through a break up in a relationship.

Duration of Action

The final element within the core of the transformation cycle is the duration of your actions. This is the key ingredient that separates getting 'ok' results from creating a significant change. There is no point doing everything perfectly for one day, whatever you do, it will not make a difference. All efforts need to be continued over a longer period of time.

The main aspect to consider around duration is the potential time it will take to achieve your end goal. This allows you to set some realistic time frames and expectations. You would also want to consider the difference between how quickly you could change in theory vs a sensible expectation in the real world. This accounts for the effort of getting results week after week. There are different time scales for losing body fat vs gaining muscle or changing behaviours.

It is also helpful to be aware of the time it takes to see the first initial changes in any area. The sooner you know you are on the right path the better. It gives you that early positive feedback that your plan is working or a warning that you need to change something to get results.

Losing Body Fat

You can normally see a body fat change within 5-7 days of eating less food than you need. As you may be awful at seeing your own body change then perhaps it will be take a couple of weeks to notice progress. The early stages of body fat losses are rarely from your worst areas but if you look in the right places it is noticeable.

Some realistic changes in body fat would be between 0.75-1.25% body fat lost per week. This higher range is very hard to sustain for many consecutive weeks.

In correlation to your clothes, they will feel a bit looser 7-10 days after last trying them on. This is assuming the clothes you used measure both your upper and lower body, as you do not know where your fat will be taken from.

If you are going to use weight, you could expect to see around 0.5-1% of genuine weight loss per week. It is very hard to impossible to work out what is genuine loss vs water loss due to the many factors that make weight so unreliable. Weight loss at more than 1% of your body weight is hard to sustain.

If you are going to be using weight as a measure then taking it every day and averaging the scores across a 7 day period is the most reliable method to compare week on week data.

So if you are 70kg, you could expect losses of between 0.35 to 0.7kg /week, or at 100kg that would be 0.5kg to 1kg a week of genuine fat loss.

If you were to look at these rates of change over a longer term you could say that you expect to lose 4% body fat in a month or 10% body fat over three months. If you lost 4% body fat you would find all your clothes are looser and everyone has noticed you have lost body fat and look thinner. A 10% fat loss is a spectacular transformation and you would typically lose 2 dress sizes (e.g. 14 to a 10) or 4 inches off your waist size for men (36" to a 32").

For a 70kg person that would be 1.5 to 3 kg of genuine weight in a month and in three months 4.5 to 9kg. In addition, this will often show as even more on the actual weighing scale. For a 100kg person this would 2-4kg within a month and 6 to 12kg in three months of genuine losses.

*** The above scenarios are really quick!!***

Due to crazy internet marketing, massive weight shifts from water loss in low carb diets and the odd crazy person who lost so much weight you couldn't believe[34], almost everyone has the wrong perception about their potential speed of progress. If the above sounds slow then you just need to multiply these results by four to see what that means for a year.

At the above speeds you would have lost 40% body fat in twelve months!! Hardly anyone on the planet has that much fat to lose. You would drop 8 dress sizes, as in dress size 22 to 6 in just one year. A guy's trouser size may go from a 40 to a 24 inch waist.

Weight wise, that 70kg person has now lost between 18 and 36kg of genuine weight. That means they would now weigh 40 to 52kg. The 100kg person would lose between 24 to 48kg so 12 months on they now weight 52 to 76kg. These are crazy numbers and totally unrealistic.

All of these huge numbers take most people way below their lowest possible level of body fat, weight or clothes size. Luckily the body has plenty of methods to stop fat loss happening at these speeds.

The point of these examples is to show the problems of how we perceive changing the body. These dramatic numbers over a longer time frame are perceived by most people to be really slow after one or two weeks. This is part of why you fail, you try to go too fast and then quit after just a few weeks. Even with much more modest and sensible approaches to fat loss the above shows that most people could achieve their body fat goals within a year.

Remember Your Metabolism is a Wave

In real life when looking for prolonged progress you cannot go at the speeds outlined above. Even the lowest range of possibility is probably too quick for long periods. This is because of the huge difference in the potential for your body to change compared to actually being able to stick to it.

As mentioned in section two, your body does not want you to lose fat quickly and/or for prolonged periods of time. The faster and longer your fat loss the larger the wave of your metabolism becomes. It is ready to knock you off the plan, lower your energy, take away your motivation and preserve body fat. This slows or stalls progress. The other trick your metabolism can play is to get you to respond to a fat loss period by immediately regaining the body fat back.

The solution to this is simply going at a slow steady pace or using on and off periods where you rotate between losing fat and maintenance. The main block to using these methods is your expectation. You are demanding results too quickly and you are not listening to your body during the process.

Gaining Muscle

Gaining muscle is so slow that you will usually need a month to begin to notice any signs of genuine muscle growth, sometimes even longer. You may notice faster results if the training plan activates sleeping muscles because the blood will return to these areas and stay there. This makes it appear like you have grown some muscle quickly even though you haven't. Gains in body fat can also appear as muscle gain.

How much genuine muscle you could gain is related to your lifting experience, your genetics, how well you train and the support you give to your body.

Real life muscle gains per month are very small. The vast majority of people would have muscle gain expectations somewhere between 0.1 – 0.4kg / month of genuine new gains. In three months that could give 0.3 to 1.2kg

*** The above scenario is really quick!!***

If losing fat sounded slow this appears to be stuck in a time loop. This sounds very slow but if you were to multiply this for the whole year you would be looking at 1.2 to 4.8kg of genuine muscle gains which is a huge amount.

These numbers are realistic with room for personal variation and individuality. If you were to multiply these numbers over 5 years you would have gained 6 to 19kg of muscle. That is a huge change to the body.

Too often we underestimate how extra muscle on the body looks to the naked eye. If you were a lean 57kg woman and added 6kg over 5 years it would be a dramatic and breathtaking change in your body shape. Any guy adding almost 20kg of pure muscle would be an outrageous transformation.

In reality it is unlikely you could get anywhere near some of these numbers. It is just not that easy to build muscle at this sort of speed year after year. The more muscle you gain the harder it is to continue at that speed.

It could be that you go at 0.4kg / month for three months then and 0.3kg/month for the next three months. The next year and a half you progress at 0.2kg / month and 0.1 kg / month thereafter. This would give a 5 year gain of 8 kg. This would give an amazing before and after photo.

Muscle Gain vs Shape vs Body Fat

If you think you are getting big really quickly then the general rule of thumb is you are gaining body fat. Muscle is too slow to build for you to be thinking you are getting bigger week on week. Fat is easily gained if you are purposefully trying to eat more food to aid the muscle building process. As you gain body fat you will become bigger all over and it is very hard to know if you are getting bigger through muscle or extra fat.

A reminder muscle gain does not have a linear relationship to seeing results. Muscle gain is like filling up a balloon, the last few breaths of air make a much bigger difference in appearance over the first few. The flip side to this is that it is easier to gain muscle in the early stages.

With that being said it does not take huge amounts of muscle gains to make a difference in appearance. Genuine muscle gain, especially if you are low in body fat shows up quite quickly. This is especially true when you already have a good amount of muscle, adding a few kg makes a huge change. Another element is ensuring that the muscle gained is targeted to the areas that optimise appearance.

Steroids

The numbers given are still slow if you are taking steroids. While progress is faster too many people think they will just make rapid unlimited gains when taking them. While some steroids create immediate 'fake' gains and increase size through changes in water, genuine muscle gains are still slow.

The average steroid user is just <u>not</u> adding 1 kg a month year after year while on them. In fact, many users gain hardly any muscle as they do not have the exercise knowledge, consistency, intensity or nutrition in place to back them up. Regardless of results, the health risks from taking them are still the same.

Changing Posture & Flattening the Stomach –

You could create significant postural changes depending on the issues involved within 1 or 2 months. You could notice some improvement within a week or two.

The key on the speed of posture change relates to targeting the specific needs for the body and by removing the stimulus that created the bad posture in the first place. For example, if you sit with your legs crossed for 4 hours a day or sleep with a bad pillow 8 hours a night it is very hard to undo the problems caused by this until you first remove the offending source.

More permanent reductions in creating a flat stomach and waist may take 1 to 2 months for certain issues such as a compromised digestive system. However, for more simple muscle activation related issues you can get much faster changes. You could create a flatter stomach within 1 or 2 weeks.

Noticing Physical Changes

With the above timescales for perspective you are now better equipped to know when to expect changes to have occurred and to what extent. The main two issues to consider around noticing change are;

If Changes Occurred – Obviously if nothing has actually improved you will be a long time waiting to see a change. Starting a health drive doesn't mean you automatically drop into the right behaviour pattern to produce results. If nothing has genuinely changed then you will need to change your plan or increase your adherence to it.

Ability To Spot Change – If changes have occurred then noticing them relates to how well you can perceive your own body. If you are not that self-aware it takes a much bigger change for you to be able to notice results.

I have lost count of how many people I have trained who have lost 2-3% body fat yet could not see any changes themselves. This is quite problematic as you will feel demotivated about the 'lack of results' even though you have got some. Worse still, if you continued that exact same plan for a few more weeks or months you would achieve an amazing transformation and in many cases reach your end goal.

You can improve your ability to notice changes through practice and a conscious effort. It can be helpful to have a 3rd party to act as a more objective and independent guide during this process.

Behavioural Changes

The expected speed of results with physical changes is much easier to predict than with behaviours. Physical changes have numerical formulas that you can use to calculate the possible change potential and link it to results in the real world.

With behaviour it is a different story, for every person that makes a quick change there is another person who struggles despite their efforts.

The speed of behaviour change is usually related to the number of times you do the actions that will create it. For example, if you need to do 30 runs to train your brain to enjoy jogging you could do this in 10 weeks by running three times a week or 30 weeks if you jogged just once per week.

The potential of change and what you need to do to create it varies depending on the area within the transformation cycle. Elements to consider for each area are set out below;

Motivation – You can change your motivation within minutes sometimes through having a new thought, going through an experience or simply by making a decision to start a plan.

For those stuck in a low motivation phase you can usually transform this feeling within 7-10 days. To do this you need to do some sort of action within food or exercise. The key is doing the easiest action you are actually prepared to do while feeling demotivated. This task will slightly increase your motivation at which point you can choose another action to do and then repeat this process over the following days to become motivated again.

To change your long term motivation patterns you would use techniques to develop your underlying feelings/ imagery around your goal. You would also look at its priority amongst your life and the desire you have towards the micro tasks needed for results. This can take days to months for a significant change in your motivation.

Skills Around Plans – To develop the skills around fat loss it takes a lot of attempts and repetitions which will give both successes and failures. It often takes three to six months plus to develop these. The development of knowledge is much faster but as discussed knowledge needs to be converted into a practical skill through repeated practice.

Neural Patterns – Breaking a neural pattern is much quicker than most people think, for the average behaviour you can collapse a big percentage of the connections within 2-3 repetitions and most of them within 10. This even applies to stubborn bad habits. For best results when breaking bad behaviour patterns you must ensure you address the different aspects to any connection pattern, e.g. not eating a cake may be easier on your own than when it is being passed around the office or vice versa.

For creating connections towards a new action or behaviour you fall into the more traditional habit forming advice which ranges anywhere from 21 to 70+ repetitions over an appropriate timeframe. So if you wanted to enjoy going to the gym you would need to go somewhere between 21 and 70 times to create enough positive connections. Likewise, for wanting to enjoy eating broccoli, you would need to have it in 21 to 70 meals. Aspects also apply here, going to the gym on a Saturday night is not the same as going on a Monday and eating broccoli at a restaurant is not the same as at home. As with breaking connections it takes only a few repetitions to change how you feel and to start forming a new a habit.

Stress Response – Changing your response to stress and the total levels of emotions experienced can be fairly quick or quite slow. You could see a change within a week in how stressed you feel if you implement some of the major coping techniques and/or start using a reduction method.

In general, just a slight decrease in your perceived stress is enough to increase your adherence or for you to feel different.

However, it may take many months to change your immediate or natural response to stress so that you fall back on positive behaviours rather than let it disrupt your efforts.

Changing your underlying emotional terrain or resolving the causes of stress within your life is usually a longer term project that can take many months to years to truly achieve.

Fitness Identity – Almost by its nature change within this area veers towards the slower side. Making use of ritualistic events can accelerate the identity change process. Changes in this area would happen gradually over a 6 to 12 month period and beyond. It is important to check that your thought patterns do actually update to match the latest version of you in both lifestyle and personality as they often fail to do this.

Feeling, Thoughts and Your Relationship to Food, Eating & Your Body – Your thoughts and feelings can change very quickly but will often mirror the gradual slower changes of your body and identity. Emotional experiences will accelerate change as does a having a personal insight in or around these issues. Often the only way to create new thoughts is to follow a programme designed to challenge your beliefs and behaviours in these areas. Without this kind of approach you may not see any change happen naturally.

Time to Transition Between Body Shape Classes

How long it takes to go from one body shape class to the next is best answered individually due to the number of influences. As a general guide the timescales would be as follows;

To go from a sleeper to a struggler it is not so much an issue of time but it is about the number of events you go through to change your mindset. When you decide to change you will transition immediately. The difference between the classes is simply intention.

To become an achiever most people can change their behaviours within 3 to 6 months. To get to the achiever body fat zone depends on how much body fat you have to begin with and therefore how long it will take to lose. This could be just a few months or a year plus depending on your needs.

To go from an achiever to a star performer it would usually take between 3 to 6 months for both the behaviours and body fat changes. Muscle gain and fitness development may take between 3 to 12 months.

To go from a star performer to the sports competitor class may take anywhere from 6 to 12 months, this depends on your affinity for exercise and potential for muscle growth.

The transition to bodybuilder would take around 3 to 6 months in behaviour development and 1 to 2 years for most to gain enough muscle.

The final transition to body competitor would usually take 6 to 12 months in behaviours and 1-2 years in time to change your external results. To become the top of the body competitor class, e.g. win bodybuilding shows, this timescale could be doubled to 2-4 years if not even longer. The use of steroids can alter the time scales for all muscle based classes.

This means if you are normal person who is the average struggler body type class right now it would take 3 to 7 years to transform your body through each of the levels to become a competitor in bodybuilding type shows. This is fairly fast in real terms, just 3 to 7 years to go from exactly where you are today to having a top fitness model, bikini athlete or bodybuilder physique...Wow! This is also not just about external results, but in behaviours as well. This means you would maintain the results in the long run as they are ingrained and natural for you to do.

Only a tiny amount of people want to get anywhere near the body competitor kind of physique as the vast majority just want to be an achiever in or around their goal weight. Maybe you want to be a star performer who is fit and lean in the athletic body fat range. In the real world this means you can probably achieve your goal within 6-12 months. Even if you are much further away you would definitely be able to get into this range within 12-24 months.

Perhaps you find it a bit demoralising with these discussions of such long timeframes. Maybe you were hoping for a three week blitz or an eight week programme. This is understandable as you are probably imagining a typical diet plan or exercise routine which you generally hate and do not want to follow. You are most likely also assuming you will not be able to maintain the results.

This is not the way the unified transformation plans work. It is not about horrendous diet plans, boring exercise routines or feeling hungry all the time. It focuses on finding taste, minimising hunger and having fun. It is about changing who you are and how you feel around all aspects of health & fitness. This allows you to stay that way for life once you change your body.

The Change Techniques Explained

At this point you know that your results are not based on some magical diet plan or exercise routine. Change will happen from a holistic approach using methods that alter your behaviours so you can be more consistent with your food, movement and exercise.

This chapter takes you through the most common methods you can use to influence the areas outlined within the unified theory. The diagram on the next page shows some of these techniques.

This list is by no means exhaustive. There are numerous techniques that are not mentioned here which could work on one or more areas within the transformation cycle, e.g. hypnosis or metaphor based therapies. It is beyond the scope of this book to outline every possible technique. All the methods discussed here are designed for you to be able to easily do on your own at home.

In section 4 you will find plans that use these methods such as the 26 week 'Master Plan'. Within this you will see many different examples of the techniques. You can also learn more by downloading the book bonus material at www.benwilsonuk.com/bonus

The Grand Unified Theory of Weight Loss

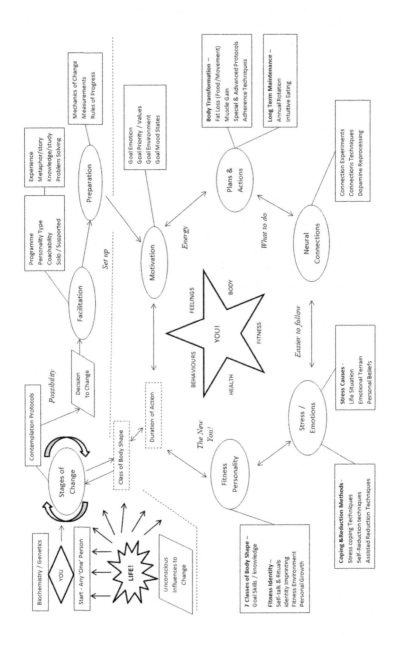

Stages of change

To accelerate how quickly you make the decision to change you can look at ways in which you consider your goal and what is needed for you to commit to taking action.

Pre-Contemplation Protocols

This is a difficult step to develop because the person is not actively committed yet or even has a target. If you have read this far then for sure you will either already be in action or in the next stage of contemplation.

However, you may have people in your social circle who you would love to wake up and kick start them into being healthier. This is an area that needs more research but as a general strategy you would need to cycle through the following three sources and provide different stimuli until they move to the contemplation stage;

Belief Building – You should be eroding away negative beliefs like it is impossible to lose weight, it is too much effort or that they are not the type of person who can get results etc. The goal is to increase the level of belief about how change is possible and that they are the kind of person who could do it.

This can be done by giving examples of people with similar life circumstances or demographics who have been successful. You could also ask questions around the limiting beliefs, e.g. if they think it is impossible to lose weight you could ask; what would happen to your body in a famine? You could recall examples of moments in their life they have lost weight or did a great job in another area of life that required changing their behaviours and commitment.

Agitation of Pain – The person needs to feel pain and annoyance around their current situation. You could ask about how frustrated they feel with their energy levels or the fit of their clothes etc. You can also get them to imagine what their future holds if they do not make any changes, you could ask; 'Where do you think you will be in 5 years with your health, fitness or body on your current trajectory?'. Other methods could include seeing a current photo or trying on an item of clothing to find it no longer fits.

Create a Positive Association to Change – The process of change needs to be a good thing. To help this you would need to downplay the negative elements and increase the good feelings around change. Showing examples of those who got results while <u>not</u> doing the things that puts the person off can help greatly, e.g. look at this woman who lost weight while still eating a bit of chocolate every day. Discussions around the good feelings of their goal would also be helpful, when did you feel your best with your body? How would you feel if you were at goal weight? You may need to emphasise a slow easy start to make it more appealing to begin.

*****

It is important to provide all three elements as a stimulus. If they have no belief that change is possible yet you agitate the pain of their current situation they will not take action, they will just feel despondent. Even with the pain of the current situation aroused if the tasks they think they need to do sound like the worst thing imaginable it will not be enough to even contemplate starting a plan. Due to these factors interplaying with each other it is better to cycle through all the methods so they can bounce off each other and generate momentum. One issue with this stage is getting people to emotionally engage in any part of the process. They may not answer your questions or only superficially consider them.

Contemplation Protocols

The main difference between this area and pre-contemplation is that you are now active in the process. The best way to accelerate this stage is to rotate through the three inputs of building belief, agitating pain and associating positivity to change.

Pain and frustration at your current or likely future status are usually the best motivators for you to commit to change, albeit it still needs to be done alongside the belief in results and a positive impression of the general process involved.

The easiest way to consider these elements is to answer questions such as those set out below. You can also look at relevant parts of this book such as the beliefs of impossibility in section 1 etc.

Remember that this part of the process is about making a decision to change and not working out the details of how you will create that change. Those are covered in the facilitation segment.

Questions to use within this stage are below, for best results you should discuss your answers with someone else or failing that, write them down so you can see them on paper.

Belief Questions –

-What would happen to your body fat levels in a famine?
-How many times have you lost body fat previously?
-How long have you sustained previous body fat levels for?
-What good behaviours have you developed previously in life?
-What bad behaviours have you stopped doing previously?
-In what other areas of your life have you been successful?

Agitation of Pain Questions –

-How would you feel if you were the same or worse at your next landmark birthday?
-What would be the consequences if things were to get worse going forwards within your goals areas?
-Who would you not want to run into or meet because of how you are currently?
-What are you missing out on by not achieving your goals?
-Who also suffers in your life as a consequence from your lack of success in this area?

Creating a Positive Association to Change –

-What one or two things are putting you off most from committing to change?
-What expectation is putting you off from taking action?
-Who is putting you off from deciding to change?
-How could you get started without any of the negatives that are putting you off?
-What is the smallest action you are prepared to do today?

Facilitation

After making the commitment to change the facilitation stage is where you will work out the best route forward. There is a skill to this in that you want to ensure you have the right approach from the start but at the same time you want to take that first step as soon as possible. It is common to see people get stuck in this stage for months or even longer.

To do this part effectively and quickly you simply need to sit down and think about the key areas around setting up a plan. This can be done by answering the questions below, ideally discuss your answers with someone else or failing that write them down;

Programme Structure –

-How does your plan account for behaviour change and the behaviour patterns behind your eating or movement?

-What programme, group or coach could be part of your transformation and in what capacity?

Personality Type & Individuality –

-What can you learn from previous successes to apply now?

-What can you learn from previous failures to apply now?

-How does your approach account for the different learning styles? (Personal experience, problem solving, metaphor & story, knowledge & learning)

Coachability –

-What should you do if you are not on making progress?

-How will you focus on changing who you are as a person?

-How are you taking a long term approach to getting results?

-What are you not prepared to do?

Taking That First Step –

-What elements are putting you off the most from starting?

-What have you always wanted to try or experiment with?

-What is the simplest and easiest way to start today?

*****

Use these questions as a guide to work out an effective plan to move forwards. If you are currently doing a plan then you can use this same process to evaluate how well it fits your needs. From this you can make additions or changes to your approach. How to integrate your current plan with the unified theory is outlined in section 4.

Preparation

The goal of the preparation phase is to establish efficient fundamentals which will allow for the process to run smoothly. There are three main areas.

Mechanics of Change – This is developed initially by some old fashioned learning via reading or studying. Section one and two took you through that process. You can also develop your knowledge by combining it with your personal experiences. You will want to be very clear on how physical change happens otherwise it makes getting results much more difficult.

Rules of Progress – To develop this aspect you can begin by answering questions to understand your current patterns around how you evaluate your effort and progress.

To put in place more efficient beliefs in this area you will need to use conscious and focused practice. It can be helpful to use a third party to guide you with this. An example of this exercise can be seen in the 'The Master Plan' in section 4.

Measurements – The way to establish an effective measurement system is through practice. Initially you will need to focus on how to take the first set of measurements. Thereafter you will refine your skills through taking regular re-measures and paying attention to how the various traits change. Over time you will develop your abilities around self-evaluation and consistency in tracking progress.

*****

With these in place you will be well set for progressing forwards. It is important also to keep an eye on all of the above fundamentals as sometimes you will drift back into old unhelpful habits.

Motivation

There are various techniques used within the four main motivation areas aimed at increasing both the magnitude and consistency of your motivation levels.

Goal Emotion Methods

These focus on evoking desire and emotion within you towards your goals. This is done mostly through using different types of visualisation. The more emotion you feel the more energy you will have towards your goals. Exercises you can do include:

Visualisations – This refers to spending time thinking about what feelings, benefits and successes your goals would bring. It could be that you sit down for five minutes every evening or perhaps you spend a minute before every exercise session focusing on why you want to achieve your goal.

Everyone has the skills to do a visualisation as it is nothing more than a combination of using your imagination, remembering moments from the past and / or thinking about what you want in the future.

Through imagining the potential outcomes you will produce real emotions within your body as you do it. This can drive your actions going forwards. Most athletes use visualisation techniques of some sort due to their benefits.

Dickens Pattern – This method directs your visualisation to look into the future at the consequences of success / failure around your goals. It has you imagining potential scenarios both in the short and long term. The name comes from the story of 'A Christmas Carol', by Charles Dickens, where scrooge is taken on a journey of his potential future.

To do this you would dedicate some time to think about how your life would look across all areas if you failed to make any progress or regressed with your body. How would your life look in 6 months, 1 year or many years into the future?

Following this you would then consider how being successful in your goal would look across your life in 6 months, 1 year or many years into the future. You would repeat this regularly.

It is a powerful technique as you are able to see what your life will look like in years to come depending on your results. It is good for creating urgency as you can see the consequences in the future for your failure to take action now.

*****

There are a large variety of visualisations and different exercises that come under the two classifications above. The key to all of them is frequency. The more often you use any of the above techniques the more likely you are to imprint the feelings into your mind-body. This will make it more available to help you through the times you need extra motivation. Too often people worry about if they are doing the exercises right rather than simply putting in the repetitions. If you do them enough you will end up doing them well.

The other key element alongside frequency is engagement. You need to mentally engage with the process. You may try putting a motivating photo in a prominent position but this usually does not work. This is because it never creates any engagement. All motivational techniques need to create some level of mental activity and/or encourage you to take action.

These goal emotion techniques will imprint your goal image into your mind and increase motivation. You will want to link this motivation to doing the key actions that brings results.

Goal Priority Methods

The emphasis here is on ensuring that your goals in health and fitness are not swamped by everything else that life throws at you. If they can remain high on the priority list you will find it much easier to achieve great results. Methods to do this include -

Values Integration – You may believe you do not have motivation. However, you are always doing something, even if it is not what you 'should' be doing. For example, you should go to the gym but you are at home watching TV. While you could argue you do not have motivation to exercise, the flip side to this is that you do have motivation to watch that series on Netflix. We have motivation to do all sorts of things.

Values refer to what you find most important in your life. This is judged by your actions and time invested in key activities. Everyone spends their time doing something, for most it is a focus on work, family, friends and so forth.

Your main values represent a source of natural motivation. You are programmed to act in accordance to your main values. For extra motivation you simply need to ensure your health & fitness behaviours are aligned to these.

For example, most successful entrepreneurs find time for exercise because they know it makes them better decision makers and therefore more successful. Many parents discover that taking the time to look after their own health and fitness makes it easier to look after the kids and also provides a better role model for them.

You can work on this area by dedicating time to understanding your current main values and then considering how they interact with your health & fitness results.

Priority Examination - This refers to looking at how you spend your time, mental focus and energy in life and how your health & fitness fits into this picture. It includes looking at the consequences of your current priority of behaviours both in the short and long term. It also involves looking at ways to set up structures to keep your priorities balanced.

The exercises may involve visualisation techniques or spending time considering options that could work in the real world.

Micro-Behaviour Motivation – The more you can make the needed micro behaviours appealing, the less motivation you will need to do them and the more likely you will actually get them done. For example, if you have learnt to enjoy exercise you will need less motivation to choose being active over watching a film or the surfing the internet.

Much of this development happens naturally from the general plans and ongoing actions. However, you can make use of task visualisations, analysing your behaviours or challenging your connections in this area.

Goal Environment Methods

The following methods are used to create an environment which increases and sustains your motivations & behaviours.

Role Models – Through making use of other people as role models you are able to address, learn from and change the way you act in your behaviour patterns. Role models exist both in a general terms of results and specifically for certain behaviour traits. The area makes use of identifying possible role models and then finding ways to connect with them more. Simply spending time with such people will improve your motivation and consistency.

Other People – It is not only role models that can increase your motivation, anyone has the potential to inspire you to higher levels of focus. This could be people who increase competition within you or those who would benefit from your success. The opposite is people who demotivate you or reduce your motivation and consistency. You can address these influences by spending time thinking about your dynamics with other people and actively trying to culture a better set of relationships.

Fitness Challenges – When you participate in a fitness challenge it focuses the mind. Through planning and committing to an event it can greatly increase motivation over many months. There are various possible fitness challenges which come in many forms such as charity walks, treks, running events, gym competitions and much more.

There is no right option for which challenge is best suited to you. This is guided by your own personal desires and inspiration. Longer term maintenance of results is helped greatly if you continue to do fitness challenges because they keep you active and focused. You should be regularly seeking out and engaging in different challenges.

Group Exercise – A ready-made positive environment can be found in a group exercise setting. It automatically puts you around other people with similar interests. This is a powerful way to raise your behaviours levels. There are numerous options from cardio to flexibility or sports clubs and teams. You should be actively focused on discovering groups or classes which you enjoy and start attending them.

Goal Motivation State Methods

To make use of this area you will need to learn how to access the desired feelings and mood states within you. At this point you can look to pair them with the activities where you want to feel that way. This means you will be in your desired state whenever you are in that situation.

To do this you would spend a few minutes thinking about and attuning to your goal mood state. You would take note of your posture, your breathing, feelings within your body and the focus of your thoughts. To identify these you may need to remember back to times when you felt this way or visualise feeling like this in the future. You would also take note of any actions that serve to keep you in this state or will disrupt it.

Once you are comfortable accessing this feeling you can then spend a minute or two reconnecting to it any time you go into the situation where you want to be in this state. Over time you will need less and less time to access it before the event with it eventually becoming automatic.

Another element to this area is being able to break out of a negative state as soon as possible. This is mostly developed through doing it in real life. Many of the strategies around how to handle lower motivation periods while following your plans are based on breaking you out of a negative mood state.

It can be helpful to role play and practice what you could do to edge yourself out of this state, so you are prepared for when it happens in the real world. In general you will need to move your body and change your actions in some way.

Plans & Actions

There are various different plans and elements to use. These all fall under the banner of a unified transformation plan, which includes every element within all of the plans. The main components parts of it are outlined below.

Body Re-Composition Plans

These protocols are designed to change your body by focusing on the main physical inputs, including;

Movement Plans – This refers to focusing on how much activity you are doing in general life. This may be how many steps you are walking or how much time is spent commuting to work on a bike etc. This is not a formal or traditional exercise programme. It is about being more active in life. This could involve setting a target step number or amount of time that you are active per week.

Exercise Plans – These are formal plans to follow to develop your fitness and muscle. This can also include movement done via exercise. It is essential to use a formal exercise routine if you are looking to build muscle or develop your fitness to any great extent. The programmes will outline when to train, what to do and how to develop your training from month to month. Overtime as you become fitter the protocols will adapt to match your improved abilities.

Sensible Eating Plans – These approaches are based on using very simple principles around food and eating. There is no right or wrong on what should be included under a sensible approach but the focus is on being 'good' while staying away from being too extreme or imposing heavy restrictions within your eating scheme.

'Healthy' Eating Plans – There are various schemas of healthy eating you may choose to follow including clean eating, low inflammation diets, food eliminations strategies, being vegan or vegetarian and much more. This would also include intermittent fasting and low carb / keto approaches.

Calorie Controlled Plans – Many people prefer to address their nutrition through a calorie controlled approach. This may mean you just eat what you want and ensure you hit your calorie numbers or in combination with the previous plans. This would also include diets based on using macros.

<u>Nutrition Plan Details</u>

The key to all of the above approaches is not so much the plan but how you tailor the details of it to your needs. It is your adherence to any strategy that gets results. To improve your ability to stick to it considering the following:

Taste – Perhaps the biggest and most important element is getting enough taste in your diet so you can follow it. The search for taste should be the most important priority of any nutrition schema. The key is how you increase taste without dramatically increasing the amount of food you eat. This comes from experimentation and working on your cooking skills and knowledge.

Logistics vs Lifestyle – The plans you use have to be able to fit into your lifestyle and still work during stressful periods. If you have to prepare all your meals one week ahead then how do you stick to this if you are travelling or busy with work? Your plan needs to be adaptable to the circumstances that life can throw at you. This could mean having a secondary approach available or being more relaxed within certain elements.

Your Body's Reactions – The body gives out signals after eating but we do not usually notice them. Following every meal you will get feedback in terms of hunger, energy, mental focus and more. These are related to the size of the meal, the macro ratios and the types of food you ate.

There are also signals day to day about how the food schema is helping or hindering the body. These signs should be used to adjust and optimise your plans.

Adherence Techniques – There are other strategies that can be used for adhering to a plan, especially under more difficult conditions. These focus on making it easier and more appealing to move, exercise or make better nutrition choices.

<u>On – Off Periods –</u>

A key element of the unified transformation plans is that there are periods of fat loss interspersed with periods of breaking even. This on/off approach is essential for long term maintenance and also being able to follow a plan long enough to get results.

The on/off periods can be structured and planned into the approach or just come as a side effect of living life, e.g. going on holiday for a week. If you do not structure in these periods your body will naturally lower your adherence over time. This is often subtle and appears to happen because of events in your life rather than your prolonged dieting, e.g. you have a bad week of eating because of stress but if you had taken a rest from fat loss this same stress would not have disrupted your efforts.

*****

All of these above technique can be used to create your body re-composition plan.

Behaviour Change & Influencing Plans –

These approaches are focused on developing new behaviours or on increasing the likelihood you will act a certain way in different situations. They can be worked on alongside the body re-composition plans or done instead of them depending on time, energy and priority.

Behaviour change approaches are usually followed for a short period of time to focus on one or two specific elements. The different types of methods used in this category include;

Neural-Connections Plans – These focus on changing your food or exercise patterns to influence your neural pathways. There are many different possible behaviour experiments and how they are put together depends on your specific needs and connections to improve.

Behaviour Techniques – This refers to the many types of exercise used within the transformation cycle. This includes the methods for increasing motivation, reducing stress and so forth. A technique may be used for a short period of time or worked into your schedule as a regular part of your routine.

Special Protocols – This links into plans for addressing binge eating patterns, working on body image or developing your intuitive eating skills to retrain your natural eating. These do not need to be done by everyone but for those who need it they be transformational. The specifics of these plans are beyond the scope of this book.

Long Term Maintenance Plans

This draws upon the elements seen in the previous approaches. The aim is to do the minimum amount of tasks needed to maintain your newly achieved goal body.

In practice this means putting in place certain periods for fat loss during the year, e.g. the first week of January to lose the weight gained over Christmas. There are also protocols you can do at other points during the year to keep your neural connections in check. It is very simple to maintain your body if you do these things.

Actions

It is easy to get intimated with all this talk of different plans, methods and techniques. However, every plan of any sort comes back to your actions. There are various simple actions that can transform your results. You will see some of these in the plans in section 4. Perhaps all you need to do is tune into how you feel after eating, start using a stress management technique or spend a minute focusing on your goals every night. This one action may set in motion the process to produce a fundamental change in your results. It can be as simple as that!

Neural Connections

The only real way to change your connections and associations is through <u>doing</u> something different and then repeating the action enough times. This will form a new connection or scramble the unwanted old one. Training your brain is a numbers and repetitions issue and if you let the number of actions be your measure you will do well.

Behaviour Experiments

These are designed to retrain your neural pathways around one particular facet of your behaviour. A behaviour experiment is when you consciously change your actions for a short period of time, e.g. you leave a little bit of food on your plate every time you eat for a few days. The secret to success with these is that you focus on only one facet of your behaviours, if you do this almost everyone can complete any challenge.

It is when your attention is split from trying to do more than one thing that most people run into problems. For example, if the goal for the day is not to eat during the afternoon (to retrain your natural hunger patterns and snacking habits), then you do not need to worry about anything else, e.g. eating healthily, avoiding sugar or limiting how much you eat. Just focus on the one facet for that day which is not eating in the afternoon. Likewise, you can begin any experiment slowly and gradually by starting only a little outside of your current comfortable behaviour patterns. You can see a few example behaviour experiments in the programmes set out later.

How Many Times to Do the Tasks

For the average person each of the tasks takes some mental focus the first time you do it. After doing it though, you will probably be surprised that it was easier than you thought and different to how you expected it. Each time you do it you will find it becomes easier and easier to do. Some tasks which work on strong connections may need many repetitions until it is totally comfortable. For many other tasks you can create a change very quickly in just few attempts.

In general most old 'bad' connections can be broken between 3 and 10 repetitions. Forming new 'good' connections it is a little slower, 10 repetitions will create a change in the feeling towards the task while it may take anywhere from 20–70+ reps to create a full on habit where you do not need to think about doing it.

Safety and Common Sense

Some of the tasks involve not eating for a short period of time or changing your exercise protocols. For some people, they may initially be very sensitive to changes in their eating or exercising patterns. If you happen to feel dizzy or suffer any negative side effects then stop the experiment and go more slowly into the task.

It is not a race to get the tasks done. It is about training the mind and body to be fundamentally different going forwards. The overarching theme is to use common sense and not to be so competitive or stubborn that you lose perspective. There are no medals for pushing through pain in this area, just stop and come back another day. You will still get great results if you are sensible and patient with the process.

Dopamine Reprocessing

The most effective way to address this area is based on your underlying needs. The main approaches include;

Dissociate From Simple Dopamine Eating Triggers – The simplest level to address dopamine is through your environmental cues triggering you to eat. This could be having to eat a certain food after dinner or needing to eat at specific time of the day. The behaviour experiments outlined above achieve most of these goals, e.g. not eating between meals, gentle fasting experiments etc.

Dissociate From Food Based Dopamine Triggers – Other times you will need to specifically go after the connection between food and dopamine stimulation. This may involve removing all the main offending foods for a period of time. This will allow you to become more sensitive to those foods again. This could be a two week sugar detox, a week with no junk food, removing caffeine for 10 days or doing all of them at the same time.

Dissociate From Non Food Based Dopamine Triggers – It could be your main offending stimulant is not food or a food group but other sources of dopamine. You can temporarily eliminate the trigger for a short period of time. This may mean stopping porn, masturbation, gambling, alcohol, drugs, computer games or excessive phone usage.

Rebalance the Whole System (Dopamine Detox) – Sometimes you will need to recalibrate your whole dopamine system. In this case you will need to remove all the main sources of dopamine stimulation for a period of time. This will allow the body to rebalance the system. This involves the worst offending foods and major triggers such as porn, social media and your phone etc.

Emotions & Stress

To handle the influence of stress you will want to implement a strong set of counter measures. There are different options available to you.

Main Stress Coping Methods

The main coping methods are outlined below –

Exercise – Moving the body allows you to change emotional state and handle more stress during difficult times. The key is actually getting yourself to move when under stress. Often your exercise routine for stressful periods may be completely different to the normal plan you use, e.g. doing a walk instead of jogging or just doing your three favourite exercises and not your full programme. Any form of movement can help with stress. Dances such as '5 rhythms' have been shown to be effective in both coping with and reducing stress.

Sleep – If you get a full night's sleep (~8 hours) it directly helps your stress because you process your emotions during the last four hours of the sleep cycle when in REM sleep.

Healthy Eating – The healthier your foods during stressful times the better you can handle the challenging period. The problem comes in that your natural inclination while stressed is to eat worse quality foods. To help against this you can try to pick the most convenient and/or tasty healthy foods.

Other Methods – Any other method that does not involve food or drink which you enjoy could serve as a stress coping technique. This includes hobbies, doing satisfying tasks, connecting with friends, reading the right books, mindfulness, listening to music, turning your phone off, planning the future, helping people and much more.

Main Stress Reduction Methods

There are numerous approaches you can take to reduce your stress levels. Some of the main ones you can do alone include;

Slow Breathing – Perhaps the simplest stress reduction method is slow breathing. To do this, sit in a comfortable position and focus on breathing slowly. For example, breathe in for 4 seconds then breathe out for 6 seconds with no pause between the breaths. Slowing your breath will influence your mood and stress. You can do this for 5, 10 or 20 minutes plus.

Meditation – There are so many different forms of meditations. This includes chakra, spiritual, mindfulness or focused meditations as well as mantra based reflections. Through focusing your mind and breath you will be able to reduce your stress.

Journaling – Writing your thoughts, feelings and emotions about either your life currently or about events that have happened in the past can be very therapeutic and aid in stress reduction.

Emotional Freedom Technique (EFT) – This method involves a combination of tapping acupuncture points on your face and body while thinking about the specific stresses that are happening in your life. Through using certain speech patterns alongside this you are able to change your feelings and levels of stress around the problems you are facing. This simple to use technique works by making use of the mind-body connection within stress.

Many Other Methods – The above is just snapshot of possible methods. Check out the book 'The Body Keeps the Score' by Bessel Van Der Volk which covers extensively the methods you can use to reduce stress. Some of these can be done alone but a lot involve the help of trained professionals.

Reducing the Causes of Stress

These methods look to resolve the core reasons behind your stress, this includes;

Improving Your Life Circumstances – How you live your life and the circumstances within it influences both your stress levels and how you feel day to day. If you improve this you will experience less stress.

Often you can reduce stress immediately by making some simple life changes. Longer term you would look at setting goals and improving any life areas which are causing problems. This could be your job, financial situation, your friends, intimate relationships, living situation and more. You can improve these areas by identifying your objectives, the needed actions for change and the order to do them in.

Changing Your Emotional Terrain – This refers to using some of the emotional reduction techniques to change your total stress levels with specific reference to events from your past, your current life evaluation or concerns about the future.

Exploring the Bigger Questions of Life – Sometimes you will need to look into your own personal philosophy around the purpose and meaning of life. For many people this may merge into more spiritual questions. This can be done through studying philosophy, religion or spirituality.

Investigating Your Beliefs – Examining the beliefs you hold around how you live your life and how you view stress itself can reduce it. Many stress causing beliefs come back to the interplay between "How the world should exist" vs "How it actually exists". Movements such as 'Mindfulness' and 'The 3 principles' look into this area as well as various personal development approaches.

Using the Stress Techniques

The actual process of implementing these methods would be to focus for a short period of time to learn and practice a technique. After an appropriate amount of time using the method you can then evaluate the effect it had.

This usually needs to be done when times are not so bad. It is very unlikely during a period of heavy stress you would have any inclination to try and learn a new stress management method. It is more prudent to practice and learn these techniques when you have the time and energy so that when a stressful period comes along you just naturally use them.

The stress management methods should always be done alongside a focus of trying to change your behaviours around food. The goal is to disconnect eating badly from the feeling of stress, ideally replacing it with movement. This would mean you do not need to rely on stress management methods to get results as stress will no longer act as a block to progress.

It is therefore important to work on both managing stress and changing your response to it. Be careful of thinking you need to resolve all of your problems in life to get results, this is not true. You just need to disconnect negative health & fitness behaviours from the feelings of stress.

Addressing the causes of stress is as much about transforming your life as it is about changing your body. This area requires you to take a deeper look at your psyche and make a commitment over time for personal self-growth. While it may be slower to see results in this area the changes you do see will be both profound and far reaching.

Fitness Personality

The role of the exercises within this area is to accelerate the changes in your fitness identity and thus allow them to be integrated into your personality. The exercises are also used to clarify the needs of your goals vs areas you still need to develop for continued results and success.

7 Body Classes Analysis

Your current progress within the transformation cycle can be checked against the needs generally required by each body class type. This allows you to see both the progress made so far and which areas you will need to work on going forwards. This exercise is done by comparing traits from within the classes to your own current skills.

Identity Rules Analysis

These exercises look into examining the rules around your identity and how you currently view yourself. From this you can clarify your aims in this area and the specific criteria that would constitute a new goal identity. This allows you to objectively monitor and achieve your goal.

Ritual Creation

In this area you actively focus on creating rituals to help you develop your identity and put in place good behaviour patterns. This would apply for both types of rituals:

Symbolic Rituals – You would decide what events would symbolise a transition to a new type of identity, e.g. 'I know I will be a runner if I can run 10km without stopping'. With clear events outlined you can then focus your plans towards achieving them.

Behaviour Rituals - You would look to identify possible behaviour rituals for things you could do periodically (annually, monthly) as well as weekly and daily. You would then experiment with them to ensure they have the desired effect. For example, some people weigh themselves every week or morning as it inspires them to be more active while most people find regular weighing actually causes more harm than good. You need to find what works for you.

Identity Imprinting

The focus of this method is to understand how you would act and feel in certain situations if you were already at your goal identity. The exercises involve visualising how you would be in those circumstances.

Through imagining how you would think, feel and act in the most common life situations you will encounter you are more likely to act this way in real life. Overtime this will change both how you act and how you see yourself.

Self – Talk Switching

Our words can be agents of change or keep us locked in our current patterns of thinking and behaviours. A conscious, congruent and deliberate change of your speech patterns can influence your beliefs and behaviours.

This process works by changing your words consciously to a more helpful language pattern while examining the underlying beliefs behind them. This is then added to taking action in the real world to generate more evidence and support for your new beliefs. When I am working with clients it is easy for me to challenge unhelpful mantras and slogans. It takes more self-introspection when doing this alone.

Common errors in this process includes using language that is incongruent with your beliefs, not using your self-talk in conversation and not generating evidence by taking action.

A congruent statement will contain both an element of truth and an action to replace the previously negative and limiting statements, for example, 'I'm so lazy' could be replaced with 'I'm getting more active by walking everyday', "I was really lazy, now I am getting better as I'm moving everyday" or "I am super lazy some days yet other times I am really active and move a lot". The key is which feels right and best represents both truths congruently. Ideally your language would elicit thoughts that lead to taking helpful actions and generate supportive emotions.

In my experience, this is far more powerful than positive image affirmations such as "I am full of energy and becoming more active every day". These types of affirmations are far cry from your current reality and need a very high number of repetitions to work. For most people they will never get anywhere near the amount to influence behaviour.

You can generate evidence to support your new beliefs by purposefully setting up experiments to aid this transition. For example, to build your beliefs of being in control in social situations you could start going to different events and focus on making good eating choices.

You would also want to spend time contemplating the basis of the beliefs underneath your language or any desired new patterns. In combination these steps will change your self-talk and the beliefs underpinning these.

Fitness Environment Creation

The idea of these exercises is to form an environment to ensure you are lifted to a higher level. They mostly involve other people as the catalyst of change. Methods include:

Using a Coach, Trainer or Mentor – A very powerful way to improve behaviour is to work under the guidance of someone else. This could be online or in person. Most of the best transformations have come with help from a coach in some form as almost everyone does better with support.

Types of people you could use include personal trainers, nutritionists, health coaches, sports coaches, life coaches, group weight loss facilitators, someone who has achieved your goal previously and many more. With so many options it can be wise to use various coaches on your journey at different times.

Testing & Data – Selecting some testing methods that appeal to you and booking both the initial test and retest at a future date is great for external motivation. This will create a timeframe and focus for developing the traits. You can do the test/retest yourself but if possible using someone else is helpful as it adds an extra level of accountability.

Test data could be through your doctor for your weight or a variety of health measures such as blood pressure, cholesterol etc. You could do a fitness test of some sort, be it running, rowing for cardio or strength based tests.

You can focus on your body shape through getting a body fat measurement, taking before and after photos or buying an outfit and booking an event to wear it at. Some people like to book a photo shoot a couple of months ahead.

Groups, Clubs and Teams – You can change your behaviours by being around people with a similar mental focus to how you want to act. These types of people can often be found if you join a group, club or team of some kind.

You have gym based groups such as cross fit, boot camps or military fitness groups. There are dance schools, yoga centres and walking groups. You have martial arts centres, cycling and running clubs and much more. The vast majority cater for all levels. There are groups of similar demographics such as mums fitness clubs, men over 40 groups and so much more.

Fitness Role Models – If you have access to someone who represents your ideal fitness goal then spending time with them is a powerful way to improve your own behaviours.

Your ideal role model could be someone in a similar demographic to yourself, for example Claire from the gym who is super fit and has 3 kids or John from the tennis club who still goes skiing in his 80s. It may be a dance teacher, a gymnast or acrobat. It could be someone from sports such as running, triathlon, cross fit or team sports like rugby. Perhaps your ideal role model is involved in combat sports such as boxing, MMA or karate or is a body competitor competing as a fitness model, bikini athlete or classic bodybuilder.

The more time you spend around your role models the better it is for your own behaviours and standards.

Personal Growth Challenges

These specific tasks are a powerful approach to grow as a person and should be used when an aspect of your goal needs more than just health & fitness influences. The challenges will expand your skills, horizons and/or boundaries.

There are many tasks you can do for self-development. This could involve doing charity work, studying, looking into spiritual practices, facing your fears, resolving an argument or doing a symbolic event such as throwing out old possessions.

It could mean going through an addiction programme for alcohol, sex or internet use. Maybe you decide to go after a goal area of your life such as dating again after a difficult break up. It could be you plan a travel to a place you always wanted to go or pursue a new job or career change.

There are no right or wrongs on what to do as it depends on your goals, needs and desires. You can start out with a small challenge in a particular area or go after a big challenge that excites you yet scares you at the same time. It is purely specific to you.

Global Techniques

While we have seen the main methods within each area there are some elements that affect more than one aspect.

Sleep

Perhaps the biggest multi area influence is the quality and amount of sleep you get. While we discussed this already under stress coping techniques your sleeping patterns will directly affect many other areas. It influences your motivation, willpower, calorie burn, fat processing and hormone systems. It is also strongly related to food cravings and the dopamine system.

With so many areas influenced by sleep patterns it can be a significant part of the process for achieving results. Resolving sleep issues involves a focused effort on installing good sleeping habits.

A good book on this is Mathew Walker's "Why We sleep". He outlines the significant benefits of getting 8 hours sleep verses 6 to 7 hours. Some of his basic advice for a good night sleep includes -

-Go to bed around 10pm and aim for 8 hours sleep.

-Sleep in a dark room that is not too hot.

-Avoid caffeine after lunchtime and avoid alcohol.

-An hour before bedtime, dim the lights and turn off all screens (put your phone on airplane mode 60 minutes before bedtime!).

In my experience there can be a big nutritional element to better sleep. I have seen people transform their sleep on changing foods, eliminating caffeine, abstaining from alcohol and stoping their over the counter sleep aids. I have also seen meal timing affect it, sometimes by not eating within many hours of sleeping and other times by eating just before bed.

Alongside these you may also need to use some of the stress reduction techniques to calm down before sleeping e.g. meditation, Emotional Freedom, Technique.

The quality of your sleep is also greatly helped if you ensure your mouth is kept closed during sleep. Nasal breathing significantly increases sleep quality. There are straps or tape that can be used for this.

Finally you need to also consider your bed, pillow and sleeping posture. This is very important, you spend almost a third of your life in a sleeping position so it is worth dedicating time to ensuring it is ideal for your postural needs and maximises your sleep quality.

Breathing

How you breathe has an influence on your chances of results. This happens in a few ways, for starters your breathing pattern help to determine your mood states. They also affect your stress levels. Inadequate breathing can be a cause of food cravings as well as reducing sleep quality which brings consequences as discussed above. It is partly for this reason yoga and meditation are beneficial as they work on your breathing patterns.

Improving your breathing can take on a variety of methods which may include dedicating time to a certain style of breathing practice, adjusting your breath during exercise or short changes to your breathing to change mood state.

The main principles behind breathing to consider are;

Diaphragm vs Chest Breathing – The body is designed to breathe with your diaphragm moving downwards to push the stomach out (belly breathing). Most people breathe via their chest these days. This is inefficient and increases stress.

Nasal vs Mouth Breathing – You should breathe in and out through you nose at all times except during strenuous exercise. The majority of people use their mouth, especially when sleeping.

Breathing Tempo – We mostly breathe too quickly these days. Ideally you would be breathing around 6 breaths per minute at rest. The tempo of breath refers to how long it takes to breathe in and out. Ideal ratio for most people at rest is to breathe in for 4 seconds and out for 6 seconds.

Breathing Volume – The amount of air you breathe is also an important factor. It is a misconception that we need more air per se. We usually need to increase our breathing efficiency. This is linked to carbon dioxide tolerance and oxygen uptake.

Night time Breathing – How you breathe while asleep is a big influence on sleep quality and your overall breathing efficiency. Mouth breathing reduces both of these. There are different tapes and straps to encourage you to breathe through your nose. If your nose is blocked, assuming it is not from structural damage, it will soon clear as carbon dioxide increases in the blood which opens the nasal passages.

Breathing Methods – There are many breathing approaches you can learn that work on the above facets. I use Butekyo breathing but there are yoga breathing methods (this is much more than taking big breaths), Wim Hoff, Box breathing and much more. It is almost guaranteed you would benefit from looking into your breathing patterns in some way.

Section 3 – Summary

-The Results Process – There are many factors and influences upon why you do or do not get results and how likely you are to maintain it. Traditional methods of explaining this are out dated and ineffective for explaining body transformations.

-The Grand Unified Theory of Body Transformations – This covers all of the inputs that can affect you (any 'one' individual) trying to achieve any goal.

The starting point is your current body shape, life circumstances and personal influences such as your genetics. From this place there are a few steps to take before the transformation begins. This includes the stages of changes and contemplation protocols as well as looking at how to facilitate and prepare for the process ahead.

The core of the transformation cycle has inputs from motivation, plans & actions, neural connection, stress and emotions as well as your fitness identity. These all contribute to your behaviours and battle against the influences of living life. Over time and through consistent action within these areas you will change your behaviours and therefore your body. This holistic change inside and out will bring you back to the start of the cycle as a new person. At this point you will maintain your results going forwards or repeat the process if you have further goals to achieve still.

-Transformation Techniques – Within each of the areas of the transformation cycle there are various techniques that can be used to create real world behaviour change. These are necessary to develop you as a person and move away from relying on willpower to get results.

****

Imran, 32 – He has struggled with his weight as an adult and is currently very overweight. He used to like exercise but finds it hard now that he is so heavy. He works a job he does not like but it has some perks. He is a big emotional eater and has various issues in his life. Coming from a religious family, he came out as gay three years ago and they have disowned him.

A standard approach would just treat Imran simply as a calorie machine that needs to eat less and move more. This could be whether he tries on his own, uses a trainer or downloads an online plan. No trick, gimmick or biochemical method from ketosis to fasted cardio will work for him due to his emotional eating. After a few repeated failures he would have consigned himself to being overweight for life.

After starting to train with me Imran decided he needed to separate stress from eating. With many issues around his family that were unlikely to be resolved any time soon he couldn't change his body with his current emotional eating. Instead of starting a diet he began experimenting with the principles within intuitive eating. Alongside this he began learning different stress management techniques. I taught him Emotional Freedom Technique and he started using it most days. He also focused more on his need for sleep and started finding enjoyable ways to move his body.

When Imran reconnected to his natural hunger and increased mindfulness around eating he immediately changed his habits with food. On adoption of more stress management techniques he was actually able to stick to his plans much more. This allowed him to lose 23 Kg. On a behaviour level, his emotional eating is vastly reduced and he is confident of maintaining his results.

****

Section 4 –

Your Grand Unified

Transformation Plan

You have seen and understood the key fundamentals behind getting in shape in sections 1 & 2. In the last section you learnt how the Grand Unified Theory of Body Transformations has the potential to take anyone, including you to any goal you desire.

In this final section you will see how to bring this all together into practical action. There are plans to follow or an option to create your own program. Either way, you will discover your road map for success and how best to navigate through it.

The Grand Unified Theory of Weight Loss

The Art of the Body Transformation

Just before you look at the different pathways to achieve your goals it is helpful to understand how there is an almost artistic element to any successful body transformation.

What this means is that creativity is part of the process. Too often you will look to impose a high degree of rigidity to your routine. You demand structure and are not open to change. This often stems out of fear of getting things wrong or a lack of desire to interact with the plan or process.

There are various areas where it is helpful to have flexibility over rigidity. This includes what methods you use within your plan and how you structure it. The problem is you have had so many experts barking orders at you over the years they have ruined your confidence around experimentation.

So embrace your creativity while understanding you, like anyone, has only a limited amount of time and effort to give during any one week or month. This means you will need to prioritise certain facets which will change over time.

There is no hard formula or science to this, it is an individual approach. The ability to handle self-negotiation, to be persistent or to know which techniques to use is the art of the transformation.

You can only develop any art through practice and changing your body is exactly the same. As you go through the programmes during this section always remember that flexibility and creativity should be used when needed.

This is true for you but especially true if you are helping someone else to change, be it a friend or if you happen to work in this field. Stay flexible and creative!

Approaches to Change

With an understanding that creativity can always be applied to any plan as based on your desire/needs there are different approaches you can use. There are pros and cons with each method and example plans can be seen later on. These are;

-Structured Approach with No Formal Plans

In this method you have a set out protocol to follow so that you know what you are doing on the programme however there is no formal nutrition or exercise plans to be following.

This approach is good in that it covers the many influencing areas within the unified transformation cycle. Another benefit is that by having no formal nutrition plan you will learn how to get results using fairly natural eating. Without a formal plan it also stops you berating yourself for 'failing' when you go off the plan and ensures you get the credit for results rather than saying it was the magic of the plan itself. This is good for building up your confidence.

Some of the negatives of this method include how the structured approach is not specific to your exact needs. It is based on what most people probably need to do. Many people can also feel a little uneasy without having any formal plan to follow around food or exercise.

This is probably the best approach for the majority of people to take. It captures the ethos of the Grand Unified Theory by having all areas of the cycle contributing during the plan yet it is not locking you into a strict food or exercise regime. This allows you to avoid putting your focus on often unnecessary actions or fall back into previously unhelpful behaviour patterns. Do not be scared of veering away from the conventional approach, it has failed you many times.

-Structured Approach with a Formal Plan

This route combines a structured approach to address the different areas within the cycle while also following a formal nutrition and exercise plan.

The good thing about this approach is that you are covering all of the transformation cycle so you are increasing your odds of success. It also has a formal plan which brings structure and knowledge to the actions you need to take with your food and exercise. This means you know exactly what you should be doing.

The negatives of this approach can be that it is too hard to follow formal plans and also be able to do some of the other requirements of the transformation cycle. There are also the same limitations of a structured approach as before in that it is based on the average needs of someone and perhaps does not cover your specific problem areas enough. As you have a formal plan it allows you to 'fail' if you do not follow it and also allows you to give credit to it for your results rather than acknowledging your actual effort and actions

This method is best for those who like to follow a plan or are already following one but need to increase their consistency of results and adherence towards it. It is also ideal if you are already working with a professional but want to add in the transformation cycle elements to improve your results.

It is probably not the best approach if you are very new to changing your body or if you are someone who generally has had poor results with your health & fitness previously.

-Unstructured Approach

With this method there is no set structure to follow and instead you add in techniques from within the transformation cycle and its different areas.

This is a great method in that you can make very simple changes without much commitment on your part. If you get the right influencing area you can make significant changes in behaviour quickly which will soon produce results.

The drawbacks to this system is that if you pick the wrong influencing area you will see little benefits and likewise much of the fundamentals have not been addressed so it assumes you have these roughly in place If you want results.

This approach is ideal for someone already on a plan of action or if you are fairly good already with many of the actions needed for results. It can also be used if you have a specific issue or circumstance you want to address, e.g. binge eating.

If you are just looking to raise the bar a little or do not want to commit too much time or effort initially then this may be the right approach for you.

-Specific Personalised Approach

In this protocol the plan is set out based on your needs, preferences and circumstances. It can make use of both a structured or unstructured process as well as whether to use casual or formal exercise and nutrition plans.

The benefit of this approach is that it is completely tailored to your needs. This should mean you have the best chance to get results. You can maximise efficiency with this method so you get the most results in the shortest amount of time.

The problems with this method is that you need to be confident in knowing what you need for results and designing a plan, or have access to someone who can do it. This plan is best followed if you have access to someone who is confident in creating these plans.

How to Pick the Best Approach for You?

There are no rights or wrong answers about which method you should follow. The vast majority of people would do better using a structured approach with no formal plans, this is set out in 'The Master Plan'. It is designed to maximise the results for anyone who has struggled with getting to their goals previously.

If you have a plan or structure already in place in regards to food and exercise, or you have a coach you are working with then use 'The Master Plan +Plus' which factors your plans into the process. You can also choose this if you particularly like following plans assuming you have access to one.

You should use one of the above avenues unless you want to just add one or two techniques to your current routine to see what happens or you are able to create a personalised plan.

Whatever method you use it is important going forwards to commit to action. This is what produces results. Make sure you are open to doing things that are a little different to what you are used to doing, as this often produces the best results.

Transformation Plans

Find within the rest of this section example plans for each of the methods of approach. Everything is set out for you to easily follow along. There is a question and answer section to cover many of the main issues which may come up at the end.

There are four main types of plan in this section –

The Master Plan – 26 Week Transformation – This covers all of the different inputs upon your results done over a six month period. There is also an express 12 week version of it.

The Master Plan +Plus – 26 Week Transformation Plan – This approach covers all influencing areas but is done alongside a more formal exercise and nutrition plan.

The Targeted Techniques Plan – This approach makes use of the different strategies to develop your highest priority areas.

Your Personalised Plan – All options, inputs and structures are available to be used as you create your own plan based off your main needs.

*****

There are no right or wrongs of which approach to choose. They all have merits to them. I would suggest you read briefly through them and choose the one that feels right.

These plans are focused primarily on achieving fat loss and body composition goals. For the other holistic goals such as health, fitness and emotional wellbeing you may need to bring in additional techniques to those outlined here.

Needs analysis

Before you start your plan it is often helpful to understand the main needs and requirements you should be aiming to develop during the programme.

Your needs are influenced by your goals. As you have seen already within the seven classes of body shape, certain goals require more skills, effort, knowledge and time to achieve. Your current behaviour patterns will also dictate what you need to work on going forwards to get results.

As well as identifying your needs it is also helpful to establish a sensible timeframe for achieving your goals. Often an incorrect expectation for getting results will destroy your best intentions at sticking to your plan. It is important you adopt a longer term outlook when you begin the process. You should also be aware of when you should see the first signs of progress so that you are on the right track.

Downloadable Forms & Support Videos

For all the forms and diagrams you will see in the following programmes as well as bonus material you can download a copy on my website, to access these go to:

www.benwilonuk.com/bonus/

Use the password: transformation

*****

Before You Start Any Plan

It is vital you remove two of the big reasons you may fail before you start any of the actual plans. If not, you will be set up for failure before you ever get going. The main two blocks are an inability to chart measurements accurately and not understanding the fundamentals of change.

Measurements

There are different measures you should take to ensure you can chart progress and be confident in understanding your body. These measures are –

Goal Clothes – The most powerful measurement tool is to pick out a goal clothes outfit that represents your very end goal. This outfit should cover both the upper and lower body, e.g. jeans and a shirt, a tight dress not only a skirt. As well as your end goal you should also pick out a clothes outfit that is halfway towards your goal.

It is vital you pick out and try on a specific item of clothing. Do not use 'my work clothes', instead pick out an item from your work clothes, one that represents your end goal and an intermediate objective. Try the clothes on, even if they are not close to fitting, perhaps take a photo and write down how they feel. This will be your base for future comparisons.

*****

Using clothes as outlined is sufficient on its own as a measurement system though it is probably wiser to use a few measures. If you do not use goal clothes then you must use a selection of other measures. Avoid using just the weighing scales, which is a medium to long term statistic, as your only measurement method. It is one of the worst measures.

Ideally you would use at least three different measures to evaluate progress as every single measurement method has its own limitations, especially around shorter term fat loss changes. When taken together you will be more readily able to notice changes. Other measures could / should include:

Circumferences – Your limb size is a good way to chart changes. You can easily measure your neck, chest, arms, waist, hips or legs using a tape measure. Stomach measurements need to account for bloating which can vary greatly for some people and is affected by many things such as simply eating a large meal.

Photos – Before, during and after photos are powerful. Especially for showing you how much you have changed since the first day. They can also act as a good motivation tool for preventing you going back to where you started when you have achieved your end goal. Photos should be taken both in your underwear and your goal clothes outfit.

Body Fat % - Using calipers or electronic scales will give a direct measure of your body fat. The score you get is good for charting progress month to month but not so accurate for week to week changes. This is because your results can vary due to the tester or the scales being inaccurate (they are affected by hydration). Typically the electronic scales also only measure your body fat in the lower body which undermines accuracy in charting whole body changes. This measure should not be used on its own for charting progress.

Weight - For most people they would do better if they didn't use weight and instead stuck to the methods outlined previously. Alternatively, it could be that you take your weight at the beginning and very end of the transformation only.

If you do want to use weight it is often best done by weighing yourself daily and comparing your 7 day average of results. This eliminates much of the variety you will see. Some women may only be able to compare weekly data with the same week/stage of their last menstrual cycle for consistency.

Weight should not be used as your only measure for charting progress. You should also avoid it if you find it demotivates you or you have an unhealthy relationship to it from before. Ensure you are able to resist the temptation to evaluate progress on your daily changes, instead only use your 7 day average for making conclusions about your data. If unable to do this then consider not using weight at all as a measure.

Lines of Shadow / Vascularity – Other signs of body fat loss includes seeing veins on your body or lines of shadow in the muscle. These will increase as you lose weight and you may notice yourself becoming more toned or bonier. You may also feel your rings and watches becoming looser and shoe size decreasing. It is important to look all over the body for improvements and not just at your worst areas.

General Feel – Your general feeling will also indicate how body fat is progressing. Though it is open to interpretation it works well for most people. Be wary of variations in mood, e.g. most people would rate themselves higher in body fat after eating some cake or drinking alcohol because they feel guilty or sluggish even though their body fat is the same.

Other People's Comments – As you progress people will begin to comment on your fat loss. This, like the weighing scales, is a medium term measure as few people will notice your day to day changes, especially early on. In general, leaving your progress open to others evaluation is of course an awful idea but it can be a small contribution to your evaluation alongside the other measures above.

For goals that do not involve body composition changes then it is also good to get a measure before you start. The main ones you may use are –

Health Measures – This can involve medically administered tests, e.g. blood pressure, cholesterol or you can evaluate how a specific health traits changes, e.g. energy, skin. With my clients I use a 'Health Traits Evaluation Test' which surveys all the different aspects of your health using a self-rating scale. You can download a copy on my website.

Wellbeing & Emotions– These can be measured by simply gauging your own feelings within the different areas and then re-evaluating them periodically. This may refer to your confidence, happiness, energy, emotional stability etc.

Fitness Measures – There are various fitness tests you can take to monitor the different elements of fitness, e.g. 5km run, strength tests etc. With my client I use a Fitness Profile Test which is a comprehensive evaluation of all the different fitness areas.

Re-Measurements

There are no rights or wrongs on when to remeasure. In general you should try your goal clothes on every week, regardless of expected results (avoid only measuring when you know it will be positive). Other traits such as body fat percentage and circumferences should be taken every few weeks as changes are unreliable week to week. Photos would be done every 1 or 2 months. Weight, if used at all, should be taken every few weeks or if you insistent on using it then take daily and compare your 7 day average week to week. This is better than comparing just your Monday to Monday score.

For non-body composition measures you would retest ever few months due to the slower timescales that they change.

Results Expectations & Timescales

Whatever approach you take it is important to understand realistic timescales. You cannot cheat the system, if you need months to get to your goal then accept it will take this time. Patience is an important part of the process.

The other side to this coin is to understand you do not have to wait eight weeks to see changes. With a full battery of different tests you would expect to see small changes within five to ten days in regards to fat loss. Other changes such as energy, how you feel and so forth can be even sooner.

It is really important you are open to seeing changes and not going to downplay or try to undersell what you see. When it comes to measurements you want to be neutral, clinical and as factual as possible.

While I would implore patience around results in that it is never as fast as you would like, results are also much quicker than perhaps you expect. This is because you probably underestimate how even a fairly small amount of progress will change how you look and feel about yourself.

Real Life Measurement Issues

An ongoing issue around noticing change is how to handle good vs bad days. You will have days where your motivation is low so you eat badly and then feel sluggish and/or bloated. It is easy on such a day to think you have lost all your results and there is simply no point carrying on.

It is a real skill to be able to ignore your mind and thoughts on a bad day, to not get downbeat because your expectations have not been met or similar. There is a skill to knowing when to not listen to your own voice and when to avoid any self-evaluation. This issue affects everyone.

Understanding the Mechanics of Change

As discussed in section 2, there is so much confusion around this area. You need to know the fundamentals of how change happens and be able to release yourself emotionally from any beliefs that are not true.

The whole process of fat loss is so much easier when you understand it is about creating a calorie deficit and the behaviours / thinking patterns behind doing this. The more rules you have to follow the harder it is, for example, if you believe you need 'low carbs to lose fat' you must now not only create a calorie deficit but unnecessarily do it through low carbs. There are many different false beliefs that make the process harder.

I would suggest returning to section 2 and reading the mechanics of change once more and the frequently asked questions at the end of this section. This covers what you need to know and the common errors most people make.

It is also good to remind yourself of the process of behaviour change. Too often you will forget/underestimate the number of repetitions you need to create a new behaviour pattern.

Remember the Process

It is important to understand that the approaches and plans given here are designed to make you into the kind of person who can get results. The transformation focuses on changing you and this may take a little time. While some people see physical changes early on the majority will have to develop their behaviour patterns <u>before</u> they see any results. This can make the whole process slower to begin with but much more successful long term.

Before You Begin

Just as you are about to start your plan you should take stock of what you have learnt from your previous efforts and acknowledge your current mental frame of mind.

Use the questions below to consider these issues and to clarify the right approach going forwards:

-What can you learn from previous successes to apply now?

-What can you learn from previous failures to apply now?

-What have you always wanted to try or experiment with?

-What is the simplest and easiest way to start today?

-What should you do if you are not on making progress?

-How will you focus on changing who you are as a person?

-How are you taking a long term approach to getting results?

The Master Plan

– 26 Week Transformation

This structured programme covers all of the areas of the transformation cycle. The long duration of this plan is ideal for a gradual and sensible approach to change. It is long enough to get amazing results and it is not overly intense in regards to how often you are changing what you are doing.

If you prefer a shorter plan then there is an express version of this approach which is a 12 weeks long. It has the same content but it is condensed down into the shorter time frame. Both of these assume your main goal is to lose body fat. If you have other goals as your main target then you will need to adapt this plan appropriately.

How to Use the Plan

To begin the programme simply start on Week 1 and follow the instructions. Read the outline, answer any set out questions and consider how you will do the requested exercises. As you are go through the weeks check back into the book to see what to do next. Continue until the programme is completed.

Throughout the plan use your common sense to ensure you do not push yourself too hard or risk any harm. You will need to evaluate when to take days or weeks off from trying to lose fat. You cannot get around the issue of how your metabolism responds to fat loss. The more body fat you lose the more you will need a breakeven week or two to recharge. Listen to your body on this issue. Outside of this feel free to use your creativity alongside intuition to maximise your results.

Week 1 & 2

The first two weeks are about establishing a pattern and
ensuring the fundamentals are in place for the rest of the
programme. Do not feel any pressure to start out in in some
sort of a crazy way or that you should be highly motivated etc.
It is best to just start and allow the programme to unfold. If
you are very excited to get going then that is fine as well.

Ensure you have identified an item of clothing to represent
your end goal and take your measurements as set out earlier.
These will be used for tracking progress.

Sensible Eating

The programme starts out with one of the most effective
techniques in nutrition today; sensible eating. The fallacy that
you do not know how to lose weight is often quickly exposed
by just how many people get results by using their own rules
of eating sensibly while moving a little more.

You are the one who defines sensible, too often through a
lack of confidence or perceived confusion you will look for
others to tell you the rules of what to do with food. I ask you
to trust yourself this time, do not get out any books, ask
others for advice or make this at all complicated. Just ask
yourself what would be sensible and start to do that. Being
sensible is quite low key. For example, all of these are
considered sensible;

-You keep your foods the same but you reduce the quantities.
-You cut out a few high calorie snacks that you keep eating.
-You only drink alcohol on weekends.
-You replace higher calorie foods with lower calorie options.
-You cut in half the number of take outs you eat.
-You decide to be not quite so wild on weekends.

Sensible eating will usually not impress anyone if you tell them about it because it is just sounds like solid basic advice. Being sensible also includes not having too many rules. If you were to adopt all of the examples just given you have lost the simplicity of the plan and the practical approach.

The opposite of sensible is being too extreme with your measures. This could mean stopping all carbs, eating super low fat, going keto or only eating salad. It would include doing a juice fast, cutting out all sugars or eliminating wheat and dairy. Deciding to never drink again, removing all taste from your diet or cutting out all of your favourite foods would also be too strict and past the point of sensible. Do not try to do these even if you are tempted to do it. You can add them in later if you really want to. For now keep it simple.

In my experience almost everyone is pretty good at avoiding the 'bad' stuff when planning how to be sensible. It is rare to hear someone say their sensible plan involves McDonalds for lunch, take outs every night and snacking on chocolate bars.

However most people are bad at being moderate with their plan, you will often find your sensible approach is too extreme because of your prior conditioning about what diets should be like. It is common to find plans that are too strict with too few calories and not enough taste or enjoyment.

Steps

The simplest movement and exercise system you can find is steps and monitoring how much you walk. Almost everyone thinks it cannot be this simple and look for more exciting workouts like jogging, Hiit or going to the gym. If you are not a regular exerciser already then focus just on your steps. If you are already consistent with your exercise then add the steps focus on top of your current routine and plan.

349

This day and age every phone either has a step counter automatically running on it e.g. all IPhones have the heart/health app which cannot be deleted, or you can download an app for free. If you do most of your movement with your phone then this is good to use. Alongside this, wrist trackers such as Fit Bit, Garmin, Apple watch and many low cost alternatives can track your steps. These are better if you do not always have your phone on you.

With a measurement device of some sort in operation you can now gather a general picture of your movement. If you already have a step app then check out your weekly average for last few weeks and months. This will give you a general picture for how much you are moving. If no data to look at, then just start surveying from today going forwards.

Sensible Eating vs Steps

Being able to lose fat on walking alone is a fundamental skill. It shows the energy balance equation in its simplest form. It is also a plan designed to help find out if you are an exercise compensators. If you are one then you may be amazed by how well this process works for you as you will not be so hungry without the exercise there to increase it. You may be thinking "surely this is too simple". This is because you have been made to think losing body fat is hard or difficult to do.

The idea over time is to learn how to manipulate food vs steps to produce fat loss. To start the process, simply begin by looking at your current levels and sensibly increase it. In general, the more steps you do the better. So if you have averaged 7000 steps a day for the last month, look to increase your average to be higher than this over the next two weeks.

Rules of Progress

With the base of the plan for food and movement set up you will want to look at your rules around making progress. As discussed this refers to how and when you judge you are on the right path and therefore feel good. If your rules are set up to rarely perceive progress it will reduce motivation.

The ability to feel good for taking an action is a skill and can be practised so that you become better at experiencing it. The goal of the first two weeks of the plan is to develop this trait. It will set you up nicely for the rest of the programme. You will recall from earlier there were three main beliefs to help you feel good around evaluating progress.

Exercise 1 –

Answer the following questions about the rules of progress;

-What are your current rules about evaluating your efforts?

-What are your current rules about how you handle mistakes?

-What are your views on each of the three beliefs below?

Belief 1 - If I make any effort to get in shape or change behaviour I am progressing.

Belief 2 - If I see any positive results or changes I am progressing.

Belief 3 - If I make a mistake, I am kind & forgiving to myself as I am still progressing.

-What would you need to think, feel or know to accept these?

Exercise 2 –

For the next two weeks look to practice applying these rules around progress. To do this, review your efforts at the end of each day. Set your expectations at zero and look for ways to view what you did positively. Focus on your step movement and efforts with sensible eating. If things do go 'wrong', then work on being forgiving and kind.

Zero expectations mean anything above zero steps is progress, anything better than eating junk food all day continuously in big quantities is progress.

This is an exercise in viewing things in a positive light and in being supportive to yourself. It will involve you breaking some of your old patterns around self-evaluation. All of this will help greatly in the future.

What to Do –

Get started by simply defining your rules of eating sensibly and working out how to increase movement. Alongside this, at the end of each day take a quick review of your efforts. Focus on what actions you did and the effort you put in. Ensure you view this as a sign of making progress and feel positive about it. If anything did go badly 'wrong' then be sympathetic and kind to yourself.

Week 3 & 4

The goal of this period is to bring a little more structure towards your behaviours around food and movement as well as developing your motivation levels.

Review 1

You are two weeks into the programme so you should look to retry on your goal clothes. This is good practice for developing your skills around measurements. Take notice of any changes within your clothes or generally around your body. You would usually need to do more of the elements in the transformation cycle before you would expect to see results. However, if you have made progress it shows that you have already hit the needed threshold with your movement and sensible eating approach. If you have not seen any changes then do not worry, the results will soon come.

Setting a Goal for Your Steps / Eating

After two weeks of surveying steps and eating sensibly you can now set a rough target to aim for. Decide upon a goal seven day step average and the level of sensible eating you want to achieve. Use the table below as a guide as well as your experiences over the first two weeks. Continue your current exercise programme or if you would like to start one then pick a method that appeals and have fun with it.

7 Day Step Average	Food Quantity (Calories*)	Food Adherence Level
<5000	Very Low	Amazing
5000-8000	Low	Very good
8000-12000	Low to Medium	Good
12000-18000	Medium	Average to Good
18000+	Medium to high	Average
*Always personalise food intake or calorie amounts to your own needs.		

Goal Visualisation / Goal Priority

This task is about fuelling your motivation and developing an underlying drive. Look to dedicate ten minutes to doing these exercises every day for the next two weeks. You can also do it more than once per day, e.g. first thing in the morning and before you go for a walk. The accompanying material on my website has an audio version of this exercise.

Exercise 3 –

Goal Visualisation – Set a timer for five minutes, for the first two minutes think about the benefits of achieving your goals. Consider how you would feel on your next milestone birthday or important event. Include how others would react to you and how good you would feel about yourself if you had achieved your goals.

Following this, take two minutes to think about the consequences of not changing your body. Imagine what it would be like if you were in worse shape than today at your next milestone birthday, how you would feel around others and what would that voice in your head would be saying.

For the final minute of the visualisation imagine easily doing and enjoying the needed tasks around food and movements to get results.

Goal Priority Visualisation – Set a timer for five minutes, for the first two minutes spend time thinking about how being successful with your body helps the other areas you value within your life. Alongside this consider how not being successful with your body is currently hindering progress in these same areas.

Following this, take two minutes to look forward to the future to imagine how you would feel if in five years if you had not made improvement with your body. Consider how you would feel if you were successful in other areas but at the expense of still not making progress around your health & fitness.

For the final minute consider what it looks like when you are managing to balance the demands for your body with the other areas of your life. Visualise what giving equal priority to this area looks like. See yourself easily finding time to get your nutrition and movement in place alongside the other behaviours you do in life.

What to Do –

After reviewing your results from the last couple of weeks set some achievable and realistic targets for the amount of steps to do each day and how you will stick to your sensible eating. With this in hand monitor the data regularly to see how you are going with your movement. If you are already a regular exerciser then continue with your routine, if you want to start exercising then feel free to do it by picking a method that is appealing to you. Alongside this, dedicate time to go through the goal motivation tasks every day.

Week 5 & 6

In this period you will introduce your first experiment to train your brain around food as well as reviewing a little more of the physical aspects of how nutrition affects your body.

Review 2

Take a moment to look at both your steps over the last two weeks and your adherence to your sensible eating plan. Alongside this, take your clothes measurements and note their feel on the body. From this you should be able to see if your body fat levels have gone up, stayed the same or gone down. If you cannot tell then that counts as staying the same.

There is no need to start being negative or overly positive about the results. What this is showing you is the thresholds of your behaviours, if you stuck to 70% of your goal food and steps plan and your body fat stayed the same. Then you know this threshold of behaviours is in the break even range. It is not good or bad, simply that is what this level of consistency does to the body. Likewise, if you lost or gained fat then you can match your behaviours to the results. This is vital information to have.

If you have lost body fat, e.g. your clothes are looser than before. Then you have already established the level of behaviours to lose fat and this framework could take you to your very end goal. You just need to repeat enough of these two week blocks until you get there and adjust when needed.

If you did not lose body fat then you need to raise the bar a little, this could mean increasing the level of your steps or sensible eating behaviours. Alternatively if you did not hit your targets it is about improving your behaviour consistency to hit those goals.

Behaviour Experiment – Leaving Food

This task is designed to break the connections you may have with needing to finish a food or clearing your plate. Through years of conditioning you probably have what feels like an almost inbuilt need to finish any food or drink that you start consuming. This often results in overeating as you try to force yourself to finish a meal even when you know you have had enough. This can cause you to lose touch to your natural satisfaction thresholds.

When free from the need to finish your food you will be more comfortable eating and able to stop when you have had enough. Many people find this task to be challenging yet also very liberating.

How to Do it –

For at least 7 days do not finish any food or drink that you consume. You need to simply leave a little bit of whatever you are eating or drinking.

If you are eating a sandwich then leave a little on your plate. If drinking a glass of wine leave a little in the glass. When eating meals with many foods on the plate ensure you leave a little bit of each food type, e.g. steak and chips you would leave both a bit of steak and a few chips. If snacking on a banana or a biscuit, do not finish it and leave a little.

For those worried about food wastage just save it for later. If this is really hard then begin by leaving the smallest tiniest crumb of food and increase over time.

Food Reactions & Experimentation

You can listen to your body for feedback on how well your nutrition scheme is working. Whenever you eat, your body sends out signals and reactions over the next few hours which tell you how effective that meal was for you. Alongside this, your general nutrition schema also influences various traits which you can use for more feedback about your plan.

To attune yourself to these traits and to refine your nutrition look to do the following experiment.

Exercise 4 – Meal Reaction Surveying

For the next 7+ days tune into how your body responds to eating. To do this task simply fill in the following food reaction form at some point 1-2 hours after eating. While some traits may be easy to identify such as hunger others may be harder to classify, e.g. energy or mood, but these will develop with practice.

If you experience "Bad" reactions from the meal consider returning to the same meal again but changing something, e.g. adding in more protein or carbs, choosing rice over pasta or changing the portion size etc. You can then compare the reactions of the new meal to the previous one.

Time / Food	Reactions After Eating (1–2 hours later)				
	Good reactions	X	Bad reactions	X
e.g 7am - Eggs x 2	No hunger experienced		Hungry already / Want to snack	
	No food cravings		Craving food	
	No bloating		Feel bloated	
	Feel great energy		Too little or too much energy	
	Good concentration		Unable to concentrate properly	
	No hunger experienced		Hungry already / Want to snack	
	No food cravings		Craving food	
	No bloating		Feel bloated	
	Feel great energy		Too little or too much energy	
	Good concentration		Unable to concentrate properly	
	No hunger experienced		Hungry already / Want to snack	
	No food cravings		Craving food	
	No bloating		Feel bloated	
	Feel great energy		Too little or too much energy	
	Good concentration		Unable to concentrate properly	

Alongside this you will also want to attune to the more general influences that nutrition has upon your health and wellbeing. This is shown in your energy levels, mood, sleep and so forth. This gives feedback on your current plan and establishes a baseline for future comparisons to evaluate any changes you make to your behaviours.

For the next 7+ days review the following traits every night to compare against your day of eating.

Nutrition Reactions Form							
Rate Each Trait 0 - 10 to gauge how your food is affecting your body.							
Traits / Diet Approach	Day 1	Day 2	Day 3	Day 4	Day 5	Day 6	Day 7
Energy Levels	/10	/10	/10	/10	/10	/10	/10
Free From Cravings	/10	/10	/10	/10	/10	/10	/10
Concentration	/10	/10	/10	/10	/10	/10	/10
Emotions	/10	/10	/10	/10	/10	/10	/10
Free From Bloating	/10	/10	/10	/10	/10	/10	/10
Taste / Enjoyment of Food	/10	/10	/10	/10	/10	/10	/10
Sleep	/10	/10	/10	/10	/10	/10	/10
Other -	/10	/10	/10	/10	/10	/10	/10
	/10	/10	/10	/10	/10	/10	/10
	/10	/10	/10	/10	/10	/10	/10

What to Do –

Review your behaviours from the past two weeks and make a note of how your actions influenced your body. Adjust your food and movement targets as appropriate. If you are already a regular exerciser then continue with your routine, if you want to start exercising then feel free to do it.

You should then begin leaving a little bit of any food or drink you consume. This will train your mind to not need to finish everything you start eating or drinking. Alongside this, use the food reaction form to start experimenting with your eating patterns by seeing how you feel 1-2 hours after eating. You should also fill out the daily reactions form. Use the information from this to guide you in any changes of your eating habits.

Week 7 & 8

In these two weeks you will look to continue the experiments around retraining your behaviour patterns as well as looking at the influence of sleep.

Review 3

Look to remeasure your body fat through trying on your goal clothes. Once again link the behaviours that you have done with the way your body has or has not changed. This gives more information about the thresholds at which point you lose fat or gain fat. Use this to tailor your behaviour goals around food and movement going forwards.

Behaviour Experiment – Morning Fast

The ability to go without eating for a short period of time is a powerful skill to have. Resetting your hunger thresholds, connections to hunger and your ability to be patient around food can dramatically benefit the level of results you achieve.

Delaying eating in the morning is a good way to off-set a bad nights eating the day before or simply to reduce the hours in the day in which you eat. This makes it easier to control food intake. I found this exercise very powerful and it was one of my first experiences of experimenting with eating patterns.

How to Do it –

For 7+ days look to delay the time until you eat in the morning. Most people gradually build this process up. For example, if you usually eat at 7am then day 1 wait until 8am or 9am to eat. Repeat this over the week, increasing the delay before eating each day until you can comfortably reach lunchtime or around midday.

Listen to your body during this experiment. If you feel weak, dizzy or any negative health symptoms then break your fast. While some people can go to midday on their first day most need to gradually build up to it. It is not a race to be able to do it so just go with your feelings.

Stress Coping Techniques –

The three major stress coping techniques are movement, eating healthy foods and sleep. While we have already experimented with the first two, you would also want to investigate your sleep patterns.

Sleep allows you to handle more stress. It increases your motivation, energy, the desire to exercise and also your resistance to food cravings. The main ways to improve sleep are:

-Go to bed as close to 10pm as possible.

-Turn your phone/TV/Internet off before 9pm

-Aim for 8 Hours sleep.

-Sleep in a dark room.

-Avoid food, caffeine or alcohol if it affects your sleep

-Use a stress reduction or breathing technique if needed before going to sleep.

-Sleep in a comfortable position for your posture.

-Breathe through your nose when sleeping, use tape or a chin strap if needed to allow this to happen.

Exercise 5 – Sleep Focus

For the next two weeks make a focused effort on increasing how many hours you sleep each night. Make use of the tips above. For most people what you really need to do is to stop watching TV and turn your phone off earlier in the night, e.g. 9pm, this means you could be in bed by 9.30/10 pm and have a chance at getting a full eight hours sleep.

Ensure you focus on really improving your sleep for these next two weeks. The goal of this period is to remove the sleep debt that may have built up from prior insufficient sleep. You can usually do this within a week or two which can produce significant and immediate benefits.

You do not have to commit to this habit for the rest of your life. Think of this as a sleep restoration period to create a recharged and restored you. Removing your sleep debt can set you up nicely for weeks or months ahead. Stick to this formula on weekends as well, especially on going to bed early to get your eight hours and therefore getting up a similar time to weekdays. This is better than going to bed late and having a long lie in to get your 8 hours as it disrupts your sleep cycle.

<u>What to Do –</u>

After reviewing progress and your behaviours over the last two weeks make a note of how your actions influenced your body. Adjust your food and movement targets as appropriate. If you are already a regular exerciser then continue with your routine, if you want to start exercising then feel free to choose an exercise form that you find appealing. In addition to this begin your morning fasting experiment by delaying when you eat and gradually building up to midday. You will also want to focus on your sleep, ideally going to bed at 10pm and getting eight hours a night sleep for the next 14 days.

Week 9 & 10

In this two week block you will look to establish some external motivators via exercise to help your overall motivation as well as looking at identity as an outcome, goal and motivator.

Review 4

At this point you should now be familiar with the review process. Recheck your goal clothes, look at your general feel and retake any other measures you are using. From this you can then compare your body to the last measuring date and draw conclusions of your behaviour thresholds.

You should continue this process going forwards every two weeks for the rest of the plan. Remember measurements are not a motivational tool. They should be a neutral feedback technique to let you know how your behaviours are matching the needs of your body to change shape. They guide you in your decision process.

Goal Environment

This task is about creating some external elements within your life to provide motivation. Your environment is an underrated component of motivation.

Exercise 6 – Fitness Challenge

An effective way to boost your motivation is to sign up to some sort of fitness event or challenge. This gives you added motivation to move your body as well as directing your mental focus. There are numerous different events that may appeal to you even if you have never exercised before, examples of which are listed below. Consider which appeals to you the most then sign up.

There are many great walking opportunities. There is the Moon Walk, charity walks or challenges like the three peaks. You could just focus on training to walk a certain mountain or costal trail. You can also go on walking holidays or join groups such as the ramblers.

Running has various challenges such as official 5km, 10km, Half-Marathon and Marathon races or the free to do park runs every Saturday morning around the country. Cycling has similar events with Sportives and fun rides such as London to Brighton. Swimming has open water races and is part of doing a triathlon of course. Most of these are designed for all levels.

You can use dance as a challenge by taking up a new form, entering competitions or joining a group to do a performance. You can partake in carnival parades at home or abroad. You could also focus on preparing for weekend intensives.

There are many options for playing sports, from tennis or squash leagues to martial arts and achieving the graded belts. There are the traditional team sports which cater for most levels of ability.

There are also non-traditional sports such as rock climbing, fitness challenges such as tough mudder and similar. Focusing for a holiday is another form of challenge. It could be a waking trail like the 'Santiago De Compostela', a yoga retreat, horse riding, kite surfing or skiing.

The idea with all of these challenges is that on signing up you will end up focusing your efforts on the required fitness needs for many months in preparation of the event. This is a powerful motivator and often provides an incentive to exercise when you are not overly motivated around your body. Your first challenge does not need to be anything major but whatever you choose sign up for it now & put in the diary. Then start a fitness plan targeted towards it.

Exercise 7 – Other People

The other way to improve your environment is to be around motivating people in some form. It could be the fitness challenge you choose automatically does this or that you need to increase your opportunities to be around those who inspire you. The two main ways to do this is either through identifying specific individuals or by doing group exercise.

Specific People - Identify who and how you could be spending more time with someone who is already good at exercise or healthy eating. Who do you know who you admire for their health & fitness behaviours? How could you spend more time with them? The simplest way is to just contact them and suggest ways to meet up, e.g. a walk, doing fitness together.

Group Exercise – A very easy way to find motivating individuals is through group exercise. Some of the many possible options are given below. Which ones could you participate in?

Yoga	Body Pump	Spin Bikes	Aerobics
Weight training	Dance Classes	Kick Boxercise	Boxercise
Circuit training	Hiit Classes	Boot camps	Zumba
Running clubs	Fitness Camps	Pilates	Yoga Camps

Look to try some classes over the next few weeks to see how much you do or do not enjoy them. It is also beneficial if you are able to speak to people who inspire you when you go to these classes. Asking about their fitness routine is an easy way to break the ice if you don't know them, or chat to the teachers who are always happy to talk about their experiences with exercise.

Your Goal Identity & Signs of Achievement

This exercise is about looking at the type of person you want to become rather than the body you want to achieve. Through clarifying your objectives you are able to work out what you need to do and what evidence would confirm that you have changed. This allows you to grow into a new way of being in this area.

Exercise 8 – Who Do You Want To Be? - Your Goal Identity

Dedicate some time to think about who you are trying to become with your health & fitness goals. Look to pick out a couple of words that represent who you would be if you achieved your goal, for example, you want to become an athlete, a fitness freak, the fit mum, strong dad etc.

Alongside this consider how you want to behave and feel around your behaviours. What are the characteristics of this type of person due to how they act? e.g. a runner, disciplined, vegan etc.

This also links into groups you want to be a part of, or opposite to this, groups you definitely do not want to be thought of as being a member, e.g. I want to be one of the active mums, I do not want to be seen as part of the 'lazy people'.

Look to consider all of these elements and write down what comes to mind in terms of identity, behaviour traits and group membership.

Exercise 9 – Symbols of Achieving a New Identity

Using the labels from the last exercise, what would represent becoming this new you? For example, when I am in my size 10 white jeans I will be a 'fit mum', when I run a marathon I will be a runner, if I do not eat any animal products for a year I will consider myself a true vegan. These objectives need to have a clear line of achievement. At what point do you become a member of the different groups you have identified?

In addition to this, you should find some sort of object to represent achieving your goal. This is a symbol of your change in your identity. It could be a photo in your size 10 jeans, a medal after your marathon or you could just make up a certificate yourself saying vegan since April 12th 2018.

Once achieved, you can display it in a clearly visible location in your house. The same applies to any groups you see as part of your identity, what symbol could you put up that shows you are a member of this group?

What to Do –

After reviewing progress spend some time considering a fitness challenge you would like to do and then sign up to it so the date is in the diary. Alongside this think about how you can spend more time with other people who inspire action. Make arrangements to meet them or go to an exercise class if on your own. Finally, spend time considering the identity elements of your goal, the criteria for achieving it and what would object would represent attainment of this.

Week 11 & 12

These two weeks look to address another neural connection pathway and experiments with stress reduction methods. Ensure you start with the review process of your results as discussed in previous periods.

Behaviour Experiment – Day Time Fast

During the day there are various environmental cues that trigger you to eat even if you are not hungry. The ability to ignore these and avoid eating allows you to eat less during the day. This helpful to lose fat and can be used to eat less during the day when you have a big dinner planned that evening. This task can be really eye opening in how it reduces the likelihood you will pick at food.

How to Do it –

For 7+ days reduce your eating during the day time. Start by setting a time period that you will not allow yourself to eat any food, e.g. nothing between 2pm and 5pm. From this starting point gradually increase until you are able to not eat from 12 – 6pm. If you are enjoying this you could even extend it to not eating between 10am to 6pm assuming you can have breakfast beforehand.

Listen to your body during the experiment. If you feel weak, dizzy or any negative health symptoms then stop and eat some food. This fast is much shorter than the previous morning fast but it has many more non-nutritional stimuli that make you want to eat. This kind of desire to eat will disappear fairly quickly if you resist the initial temptation. This is because it is not a true hunger but it is caused by a trigger, e.g. time of the day, sight of snacks being passed around the office, making the kids dinner etc.

Stress Reduction Techniques

The goal of this task is to experiment with and practice using a stress reduction technique. There are no right or wrong options on which technique to try, the key is go with the one that appeals and to do it every day for 7+ days.

If you do 10 minutes a day of your chosen technique you will both learn how to do it effectively and be able to see how it reduces your stress levels. Pick one of the following:

Slow Breathing – Perhaps the simplest stress reduction method is slow breathing for 10 minutes. To do this simply sit or lie in a comfortable position and focus on breathing in for 4 seconds then breathing out for 6 seconds with no pause between the breaths. It can be helpful to download a free breathing app and set it for this tempo. It will then count it for you either visually or by sound.

This breathing tempo is an ideal for relaxation and health. It is common to take a little time to become comfortable with this speed but you will soon adapt.

Meditation – There are so many different forms of meditations. To do one of the many types simply go on You Tube and search '10 minute meditations' and pick one that appeals. Alternatively you can download a free or paid meditation app. Regardless of the type you choose, spend 10 minutes each day meditating. You can do the same one every day or vary between the different types over the week.

Do not get caught up in worrying if you are doing it right or if you are the kind of person who can meditate. Simply do it for 10 minutes every day for seven days or longer. At this point, after doing an hour or two in total you can evaluate the technique.

Journaling – There are two main ways to journal. The daily diary method is when you write down your thoughts and emotions about the day that you just had. It is not a work or food diary detailing what you did or what you ate, it is about how you feel about what happened today. It should cover what thoughts, worries or emotions you are experiencing.

The other method is specific event journaling. This is where you write about a specific issue that is troubling you. This could be right now, a past event or a future worry. Imagine you were discussing it with a therapist or counsellor.

You can buy a book to write in, use a word document on your computer or notes feature on your phone. If worried about privacy you can delete the text after writing it. You do not need to save them for future reference to get the benefits.

Emotional Freedom Technique (EFT) – This method involves a combination of tapping points on your face and body while repeating certain words to link into your specific stresses.

This will change your feelings and levels of stress around the problems you are facing. If you are already familiar with this method then look to do 10 minutes per day on whatever stresses are on your mind.

If you are new to this you can learn more about how to use this method in the book support videos at www.benwilsonuk.com/bonus

Week 13 & 14

In this phase you will look into the process of 'On vs Off' periods around losing body fat. Alongside this you will look into how motivational states and language influence behaviour and self-image.

On-Off Days

One of the key skills of getting in shape is not the ability to lose fat but the ability to switch out of a fat loss phase into maintenance and then back to fat loss. The only way to develop this is actually going through the process of switching between the behaviours. You have probably already done this at some point during this plan up until this point.

In this exercise you will look to specifically work on your skills in transitioning into and out of these phases. To practice this you can alternate days between following a fat loss protocol and then a maintenance plan. At this stage you should be fairly familiar with the number of steps and level of sensible behaviours with your eating to produce both fat loss and break even with your results.

With this knowledge look to do one day for fat loss, then the next day at break even and then back to another fat loss day. Keep repeating these days over the two week period. This will give you many opportunities to see how easily you can switch into the fat loss zone and then switch out of it back to maintenance without overeating. Pay attention to your ability to do this on more troublesome days of the week, typically weekends. Try your best to stick to this even over those days. It is very beneficial if you can do your fat loss protocol on any day of the week and not just Monday to Thursday like many people are restricted to.

Goal Motivation States

This task is about training you to be in the right mood state while eating. If you are in a calm, patient and contented state you will consume less food than if you are feeling rushed, stressed or have an overly excited mindset.

To feel calm while eating you would need practice being relaxed around food. The first few times it takes a little mental focus to access this state. Thereafter you should be able to achieve this feeling within 1 to 2 minutes of mental rehearsal. Through repeating this process before each meal you will create associations to being calm around food and eventually will feel relaxed whenever you eat.

Exercise 10 – Relaxed Eating State –

Before you eat a meal, take a moment to gather yourself and begin to slow down your breathing and actively relax your muscles. Imagine a relaxed sensation travelling throughout your body from your toes to your head.

Then take 1-2 minutes to imagine yourself eating your meal and feeling relaxed throughout. Picture yourself feeling calm, eating slowly and knowing that there is an abundance of food around. Notice how your hunger is comfortable and easily satisfied by eating a sensible portion. Tune into how this all feels easy and enjoyable to do.

After the visualisation you can now start to eat your food. To aid calmness, look to consciously slow down your eating. This is helped if you put the fork down after each mouthful and chew thoroughly. While eating, think or say to yourself, "I feel calm" and "I can eat later if I need to, I will just eat what I need now". (Edit or use any other phrases you find helpful)

Do this visualisation before every meal for the next 7+ days.

Self-Talk Switching –

Your language can keep you stuck in your current patterns or open up an avenue for change. This exercise is about adopting new self-talk or mantras to help you get results. Changing your language happens through modifying your self-talk while challenging your underlying beliefs though action and contemplation.

Exercise 11 – Changing Your Self-Talk

Follow the different stages in this exercise to integrate the new language patterns into your psyche.

Identify Helpful Mantras – The following mantras and beliefs will generally help you during the weight loss process. Pick out 2 or 3 that you would like to encompass;

I can achieve my goals	- I can change my behaviours
I can lose body fat	- I can maintain my results
I can easily miss a meal	- I can leave food on my plate
I eat what I need then stop	- I stop eating when I feel full
I enjoy moving my body	- I move my body everyday
I like exercise	- I am confident exercising
I have good self-control	- I am motivated
I am calm around food	- I am relaxed when eating

-I can eat sensibly in social situations
-I am ok with doing a short or easy exercise session.
-I can enjoy social events without alcohol.
-I find ways to handle stress in a healthy way
-I am adaptable within my health & fitness behaviours

Create A Congruent Statement – Develop a congruent and supportive statement to replace the above mantra to use while you change your beliefs. For example, I like exercise – I sometimes like exercise, or I like exercise the more I try different types. Alternatively, I can easily miss meals – I have missed meals in the past without any problems, or I am slowly increasing the time I can go between eating. With your congruent statement created you will want to use it within your internal dialogue and in conversation.

Identify Beliefs – Look into the beliefs behind your chosen statements. Answer the following –

- What are your current old beliefs in this area based upon?
- What would you need to believe to adopt the new beliefs?
- What evidence would prove this belief to be true?
- Who do you know who already has this belief?

Taking Action – Plan out what actions you could do to support the development of your new beliefs. This may be a series of tasks, for example, to help with 'I move everyday' you could do 21 day exercise challenge.

Developing the process – Your beliefs and self-talk develop as you generate more evidence from your actions. Update your words and behaviours to match this until the new beliefs are cemented. For example, I sometimes like exercise may become I mostly like exercise.

Continue Over Time – Once you have developed your language and beliefs on your chosen mantras you can return to this to pick another element if needed.

Week 15 & 16

These two weeks continue the previous work done on creating better connections and discovering stress techniques that work for you.

Behaviour Experiment – Evening Fast

The ability to go without eating for a short period of time is a powerful skill to have. Being able to stop eating early into the evening and not eat for the rest of the day can be used to counteract having a big lunch or eating too much during the afternoon.

How to Do it –

For 7+ days gradually reduce the time at which you stop eating in the evening, for example, no eating after 9 pm, then a couple of days later no eating after 8pm and so forth until you can comfortably not eat after 6pm. Listen to your body during any food elimination. If you feel weak, dizzy or any negative health symptoms then break your fast.

It is vital you move your usual evening calories earlier into the day so you have eaten enough food by 6pm. It is common to see people eat 50% of their food at night. You therefore need to move that food earlier in the day before the cut-off point. If you fail to do this you may end up really hungry.

The evening usually has the most non nutritional reasons to eat. This means you may get various desires or cravings. Assuming you have eaten enough food that day they will disappear soon afterwards as they are not genuine reasons to eat. Therefore look to sit through them as they will get less and less the more you do this exercise.

Stress Reduction Techniques –

You have already experimented with one stress reduction technique in the exercise set out in weeks 11 & 12. Look to do the exact same experiment but choose another one of the techniques to do for 10 minutes every day. Pick one of methods you did not try before out of:

Slow Breathing – For 10 minutes simply breathe using slow 10 seconds breaths. Focus on breathing in for 4 seconds then breathing out for 6 seconds with no pause in between. Use an app to guide you if needed.

Meditation – There are so many different forms of meditations. Follow along with a free one by searching on You Tube for '10 minute meditations' and picking one that appeals the most. Alternatively you can download a free or paid meditation app.

Journaling – There are two main ways to journal. The daily diary method is where you write down your thoughts and emotions about the day you had. The specific event journaling is where you write about any specific issue that are troubling you. This could be a past event, present or a future worry.

Emotional Freedom Technique (EFT) – This method involves a combination of tapping acupuncture points on your face and body while thinking about the specific stresses that are happening in your life. Used correctly it will reduce your stress levels. To learn how to use this method, check out the book support material online.

Week 17 & 18

In this period you will develop your ability to switch focus within your plan and look into your fitness personality more.

On-Off Days

You have already practised switching between fat loss and break even days in weeks 13 & 14. In this phase you will repeat the same process but this time you will do each focus for 2 days each. So do 2 days fat loss, followed by 2 days of break even and then back to 2 days of fat loss once more for the whole two weeks. Look to include weekends within this process. You should know what the protocol looks like for fat loss and break even in terms of steps and sensible eating.

Visualising the New You - Identity Imprinting

In this exercise you will look to visualise how your goal identity would act in different situations. Through imagining how you would ideally act you open up the neural pathways to be more likely to actually behave that way in real life.

Exercise 12 – Forming a New Identity

If not done so already, you will need to do the exercise on goal identity outlined in weeks 9 & 10. With this information you can role play different scenarios in your mind.

Choose 2 or 3 situations from the list on the next page. Set a timer for 2 minutes and then spend the time imagining you have achieved your goal identity and that you are in one of the chosen scenarios. Visualise how this new YOU would act, feel, think and behave. Notice how natural and comfortable you are acting this way within the situation. After the 2 minutes is up, repeat for the next chosen scenario and so forth.

Possible scenarios:

Wake up in the morning	Out with your partner
Start an exercise session	Going to bed in the evening
Finish an exercise session	When on holiday
At home in the evening	If you make a mistake
Home on the weekend	If you make a good choices
When you are demotivated	When snacking
When around your family	If you are feeling down
When out in a restaurant	When you get to work
If you are feeling stressed	While out with friends
Eating breakfast/lunch/dinner	In the supermarket
At the start of the week	At the end of the week
At the start of the day	At the end of the day

Do this visualisation for 2-3 scenarios each day for the two week period. Select different scenarios from the list above each time you do the exercise.

Exercise 13 – Creating a New Behaviour Ritual

An effective behaviour ritual within health & fitness is a repeated behaviour that enhances your overall level of consistency and therefore results. These can be broken down into behaviours you do daily, weekly or more periodically. The more of these you have in your life the more they will create a framework for you to stay on target without using mental focus or needing willpower.

Read through the list of possible behaviours you could do and look to pick 1 or 2 options from the three different areas. After doing a few repetitions of the rituals decide if they are helping you improve your overall consistency. If they are beneficial keep doing them, if not, then return to the list and experiment with other options.

Feel free to create your own ideas for rituals outside of those listed below;

Daily Rituals – These behaviours get done more consistently if you link them to a certain action or the same time every day, e.g. 7am, 9pm or after breakfast, before bed etc. Possible options include;

-Food planning, e.g. quickly planning your food for the day while having breakfast.
-Pre Eating Routine, e.g. ensuring you are in a relaxed state before eating.
-Pre Exercise Routine, e.g. focusing on your goals and reasons for exercising before the warm up.
-Morning Exercise Routine, e.g. quick active stretching & exercise routine before the day starts
-Pre Bed Routine, e.g. meditation before bed, stretching at the end of the day or Emotional Freedom Technique in bed.

Weekly Rituals – It is important to keep these weekly behaviours going even if it is a bad/busy week. This may involve you doing an easier or lighter version of the full ritual. Options include;

-Measurements, e.g. trying on goal clothes.
-Monday Behaviours, e.g. not eating certain foods that day, a morning fast to start the week, doing a run.
-Specific fitness session, e.g. training your stomach on a Friday, doing a park run on a Saturday.
-Meal Planning / Prep, e.g. cooking food on a Sunday, planning the week's food before going shopping on Tuesday.
-Self-Care Practice, e.g. an hour meditation on Friday to end the work week, turning your phone off for a day a week, socialising every Thursday night etc.

Periodic Rituals – To ensure these get done either put them into the calendar now to remind you in the future or associate them to specific dates, e.g. first day of the month, your birthday etc. Possible options include;

-Annual Health Check – Have a medical and schedule a re-tests if you have any weaker scores, e.g. cholesterol.
-Fitness Tests and Re-tests.
-Signing up to fitness challenges.
-Annual nutrition challenges, e.g. dry January, lent, Ramadan.
-Fasting, e.g. water fasts or juice fasting for 1-5 days etc.
-Specific fitness session, e.g. running a 10km every month, cycling 30 km last Sunday of the month.
-Trying on old cloths, e.g. your wedding dress on January 1st. or putting on a specific sized suit on the first day of the month.

Week 19 & 20

In this period you will look to develop your connections around other people and look more into some of the causes of stress within your life.

Behaviour Experiment – Being Healthy Around Friends

We often lose the ability to eat or drink sensibly when meeting friends or around certain individuals. This experiment is used to develop better behaviours in social situations. This task can be repeated for different friends or types of social situation if necessary.

How to Do it –

Purposely arrange a few social meet ups with the intention of eating or drinking sensibly. On each occasion eat cleanly with appropriate portion size etc. There is no need to explain why you are eating well, simply say you don't want the "biscuit/cake/drink/meal" if challenged, there is no need to justify anything.

You would usually want to arrange some easier meet ups to begin with rather than going straight to the most difficult situation with your most pressuring friends. For example, it may be easier to eat sensibly with your healthy friend for a quick coffee than a party on Saturday night. Start at an appropriate level and increase the difficulty over time. It can take a few repetitions to change how you feel around other people but it does happen in time.

The long term goal is not to always eat healthily when out socialising but to be able to choose how you want to act in any social situation. This means some days you will be good and others bad. This experiment will develop this ability.

Causes of Stress Analysis

You have looked at stress coping techniques and reduction methods already. This exercise is investigating the causes of stress. If you can cut off stress at its source it will greatly help with your behaviours. There are different ways to do this.

Pick one method to look into –

Removing Small Causes of Stress – Identify what small elements may be causing stress in your life and resolve them. This could be using social media too much, interactions with certain people or having a commitment to a club or group you no longer want to participate in. This could be something you have been looking to resolve but haven't got round to yet like clearing a room or filing your taxes. If there is an easy way to cut out of a stress source then go ahead and remove it ASAP.

Changing Your Life Circumstances – Often it is the different areas of your life being out of balance that is the cause of your stress, some of these elements include;

-*Money*: How much you enjoy your work and your earnings compared to your expenses or goals. This may include your potential of future earnings going forwards.

-*Social*: The amount of interactions with friends and the depth of your friendships. The quantity and quality of contact you are getting on a weekly basis is an important consideration.

-*Relationships:* The health of your romantic partnership including your sex life and/or the general outlook on your relationships going forwards.

-*Living*: Where you live as well as the environment or atmosphere within your home.

When any of these areas are significantly below your expectations then it can be a source of stress. To reduce these causes of stress you can do the following:

-Set out your long term goals within the areas above.
-Identify what would be a 10% improvement in each area.
-Create a rough plan for what would need to happen to achieve your long term goal.
-Create some specific action steps you could take to create a 10% improvement in each goal area.
-Go out and do some these actions steps!

Very often you can reduce stress in these areas simply by clarifying your goals and outlining a roadmap to be successful. For most people just a 10% improvement in any of your weak areas can make a significant change in your stress levels and happiness.

The key to making a 10% improvement is taking action. You may be surprised by how quickly you can improve things. For example, you can have more money by cutting out a couple of expenses or working a few hours extra a week. You can often improve your social, romantic or living atmosphere by simply changing the dynamics of how you are interacting with certain people. A clear the air conversation or chat to clarify a few things can immediately improve your environment.

Small improvements in your life situation, or even just having hope that it could change, can reduce stress enough to improve your health & fitness behaviours.

Week 21 & 22

In this two week period you will look to develop your fitness environment to aid your transition into the next body shape class as well as setting a challenge for personal growth.

Fitness Environment

There are different ways to enhance your environment, choose one or two of the main methods.

Coaches, Trainers & Mentors – Choose a professional to work with and provide support. Options include personal trainers, nutritionists, health coaches, sports coaches, life coaches, group weight loss facilitators, someone who has achieved your goal and many more.

Groups, Clubs and Teams – There are many types of groups which allow you to meet and spend time with people on a similar wavelength. You have gym based groups such as cross fit, boot camps or military fitness groups. There are dance schools, yoga centres and walking groups. There are also non-exercise local healthy living groups on websites like Meetup.

Testing & Data – Select some testing methods that appeal to you. Book both the initial test and retest test at a future date. This could be a health check with your doctor, a body fat measurement, fitness test, a photo shoot or buying an outfit for an event.

Fitness Role Models – If you have access to someone who represents your ideal fitness goal then spend time with them. You can ask to train together or for them to show you their routine so you can learn. Options include people in your own demographic (same age bracket, family situation etc.) or from a whole host of sports or hobbies from running to dancing to marital arts or physique competitions.

Personal Growth Challenges

These are challenges you commit towards which will aid in your own personal growth and development. They force you to grow as a person and on completing it you will see yourself in a different way through the achievement. This is important if your holistic goal includes elements that will not change solely from your body transformation. There are many tasks you can do for self-development. These could include;

-Studying or starting a course.
-Looking into spiritual practices.
-Facing your fears.
-Charity work.
-Resolving an argument.
-Starting a business
-Writing a book
-A symbolic event such as throwing out old possessions.
-Doing addiction rehab for alcohol, sex or internet use.
-Refocusing on a goal area e.g. dating again after a break up.
-Planning to travel to a place you always wanted to go.
-Pursuing a new job or career change.

There are no right or wrongs. The task to do is specific to you, your goal and your needs. Some of these tasks may seem a little scary yet you may also feel excited by them or know they are the right thing to do.

*****

What would be a good thing to commit towards doing?

What would you need to do to start towards this endeavour?

What are the main issues putting you off from trying?

Week 23 & 24

At this stage of the programme you would look to bring everything together and put out your best approach. This involves all the techniques you have learnt. Select the ones that helped the most and add them in. Food wise use the eating pattern that works best for you and ensure you hit your step target. Get focused and go after the plan as best you can.

Week 25 & 26

As the 6 month programme comes to an end you would look to evaluate your current state of the body and decide what you need to do going forwards.

Long Term Planning

If you achieved your goal already then you can drop into a simple maintenance plan. If you still have more to do then you will need to plan ahead. Things to consider include;

Simple Maintenance Plan – To stay at your goal it is fairly easy. The main thing to understand is that you will still need to schedule a few weeks a year to lose body fat. For example, most people need to do a week or two of fat loss in January to remove the body fat gained in December and over Christmas. As long as you do this you will stay about the same shape through the December/January period. The same can apply to Easter, summer holidays and stressful periods.

Alongside this you would also want to repeat a few of the experiments you have already done here, such as the three types of fasts, checking meal reactions, signing up for fitness challenges and reducing stress. Doing these periodically will fairly easily ensure you maintain your goals.

If you are not yet at your goal then it is probably because:

You Need More Time – If you have made nice progress but need more time to get to your end goal then you just need to repeat more of the same. You would have already developed many of the skills you need for success. You can extract the best bits from the plan and repeat it.

It could be that you want or need to add a more formal nutrition and exercise plan as you progress. There are no rights or wrong. You can repeat this whole plan once again or follow the 12 week Express Master plan.

You Struggled To Get Results – If you did not get great results you simply need to add in more areas from within the transformation cycle or use a more specific plan for your needs. You can still achieve your goals! If you stuck to the whole plan up to until this point you would have developed a lot of what you need for results. This means you are close to making a big change and seeing the rewards of your efforts. Do not feel despondent! It is about just adding in a few more pieces to the puzzle.

You are Focusing on the Next Body Class Type – When you have changed body type class and are focusing on the next one you need to check your progress. If you are not making great strides towards this new goal then you may need to start the whole process again to tailor your approach to the next body shape class in the pyramid. Alternatively if you are still making progress then continue with your plan. You can add in a few new techniques or elements from the next class to your current approach as needed.

The Express Master Plan

– 12 Week Transformation

This plan is the same as the previous 26 week protocol but has been condensed into a 12 week process. This means you have to do the tasks in a shorter amount of time. This therefore requires a little more mental effort and focus.

For the individual elements of how to do each step see the previous pages above. Alternatively, download the 12 week plan from the book bonus section on my website where it is all set out in an easy to follow format.

This is a good plan if you are really motivated at the moment as you will have the energy to put in the work. It also means you will cover all the areas in a shorter amount of time which speeds up the potential for a certain area or task to be able to help you. The 12 week schema is set out below:

The Express Master Plan – 12 Week Transformation			
Start	Measurements	Mechanics of Change	
	1	**2**	**3**
1	Sensible Eating	Steps Survey	Rules of Progress
2	Review 1	Goal steps / Eating	Goal visualisations
3	Review 2	Leaving Food Challenge	Food Reactions
4	Review 3	Morning Fast	Stress Coping
5	Review 4	Goal Environment	Identity Symbolism
6		Day Fast	Stress Reduction
7	On / Off Days	Goal Mood State	Self-talk Switching
8		Evening Fast	Stress reduction 2
9	On / Off Days 2	Identity Imprinting	Behaviour Rituals
10	On / Off Days 2	Healthy Around Friends	Causes of Stress
11		Fitness Environment	Personal Growth
12	Long Term Structure		

The Master Plan +Plus

– 26 Week Transformation Plan

The same structure as you just saw can be used with a formal nutrition and exercise plan. As mentioned, this is not usually the best option for most people. However, if you have a plan you enjoy, are already working with a coach or you simply like following plans in general then this can be a great strategy.

Formal Plans

There are a host of plans out there and no doubt you have tried a fair few during your lifetime. You would have seen how one plan may be the complete opposite to another. This is not good or bad, all that really matters is that you have a plan that you like and it works well for you.

There is no specific plan that you have to follow to lose fat. All plans will work if you can create a calorie deficit. This means you can eat carbs, consume fat or even eat junk food as long as a deficit is created across a week. In reality, you will find some plans much easier to follow than others due to your own biochemistry, taste and preferences. It obviously makes sense to follow the plan that is easiest to stick to.

To build muscle you will have to do resistance training in some form though this does not have to be done in a gym. The key to muscle growth is long term consistency with your training. During this time you will use various training approaches and types of training plan. This will allow you to learn more about training strategies and which work best for your body.

Nutrition Plans

These plans are usually either calorie based or guided around a specific strategy. Calorie based plans will need to be tailored to how your body reacts to the specific calorie amount. This will vary between you and other people so you need to see how you respond when doing it. If you take your calorie based plan as a starting point that is open to change and variation based on your body then this approach can be very effective.

Specific strategy plans may be based on removing suspected sensitive foods e.g. no gluten diet or focused on increasing nutrient intake, e.g. a 'clean' healthy diet. They can also focus on removing particular food elements, e.g. no carbs, a vegan diet etc. Usually these sorts of plans increase the amount of lower calorie density foods within your diet so you end up eating fewer calories overall and thus lose fat.

Strategy based plans are often much simpler to follow and healthier than calorie based plans. The flip side to this is you can still easily over eat on such a plan as many healthy foods are calorie dense and you are not consciously limiting intake.

The key for both plans to be effective is perceived taste and how easy it is to follow. The plan must be high in taste, ideally an 8 out of 10 rating for overall taste on the plan. It also needs to be both simple enough and adaptable to allow you to follow the plan during busier or more stressful times.

The final element to note is how difficult you may find combining both a calorie plan and a specific strategy approach. The vast majority of people find it too much to both count calories and apply various food eating rules. So it is better to usually pick one or the other.

Exercise

If your goals include a need to grow muscle then you have to follow a resistance training plan in some form. If you just need to lose body fat most people find exercise helps though a big percentage will find it makes them eat more food. If you want to feel good or improve your health then exercise is vital.

Whatever exercise plan you have you still want to use steps alongside it to monitor your overall movement if trying to lose fat. In most cases the exercise you do will show up in your steps. Therefore, your steps vs food intake will still determine how your body fat changes week to week. Where exercise does not show up in your steps, e.g. swimming, cycling, you can use your step count & exercise sessions vs food intake.

Resistance training plans may be done in a gym, at home or within certain exercise classes. You can use dumbbells or your own body weight amongst other tools. You will need to do at least one session per week to begin and maybe five per week or more if you have been lifting for many years and are on a bodybuilding programme.

If your goal is to feel good, most forms of exercise will get you fitter in some way, e.g. faster, stronger, more flexible etc. So experiment with a selection of techniques based on your enjoyment. Many people find moving some way every day is very powerful for mood, mental health and handling stress.

Before You Start

As outlined previously, you need to ensure you have taken measurements and have an effective system for charting change. In addition to this you need to be very clear on the mechanics of change. If either of these two are not in place it can really interrupt and prevent progress.

Week 1 & 2

This first stage is about getting into the swing of things.

Plan Calibration

These first two weeks are about familiarisation with your plan. If you have a brand new plan then you will need to go through a learning process. If you are returning to an old plan then it is about becoming reacquainted with how it works and getting back into the swing of things.

If you are already on a plan then take this as an opportunity to check you are doing it as the plan was originally intended. This is helpful to do because we will often modify and drift away from the original schema without knowing.

Exercise & Steps

If you have not been using steps before then start tracking them and take note of your 7 day average. If your phone does not have a step counter then download a free app to measure them or buy a wrist device. If you already have movement information from before you can review your previous data.

In addition to this, start your exercise programme, if new to the plan then familiarize yourself with it. If currently on a plan then recheck you are following it as intended / doing what is best for optimal progress.

Rules of Progress

Follow the exercise as set out previously for creating an effective attitude for feeling good about your efforts.

Week 3 & 4

After setting up the plan it is now about fine tuning your eating and establishing more motivation.

Review 1

As set out previously, look to review progress and draw logical conclusions on your plan verses how well you followed it.

Food Reaction Experiments

Using the structure set out in weeks 5 & 6 of the 'Master Plan' review the influence of your food on your reactions. This has been moved a couple weeks earlier in this structure than the previous approach because so many formal plans are badly set up for your body which makes it hard to stick to.

Using the forms monitor you reactions 2 hours after eating and rate your overall reactions at the end of each day. With this feedback from your body adjust the plan as necessary.

You need to have the confidence to be ok with editing your plan based on what your body is guiding you to do. Often you will not want to do this, especially if you got the plan off an expert. However, after two weeks of noting your reactions you have real world feedback to respond to. If you are having negative reactions you must experiment by changing something.

Finally you need to make sure you have enough taste within this nutrition plan. Overall it should be at least an 8 out of 10.

Goal Visualisation / Priority

As set out in week 3 & 4 previously go through the goal visualisation process each day to increase motivation.

Week 5 & 6

In this two week block you can clarify your goal steps and food structure. In addition to this you can start the process of training your brain to be more helpful around food.

Review 2

Take your measurements and once more draw conclusions about the effectiveness of your movement and nutrition plan.

Goal Steps / Eating

After weeks of surveying steps and refining your eating strategy you can now set a rough behaviour goal as a target to achieve. Decide upon a goal 7 day step average and either a calorie intake goal (if doing a calorie based plan) or the level of eating behaviours you need to adhere to (if not using calories). See previously for more information on this (week 3&4).

Behaviour Experiment – Leaving Food & Drink

Once again refer to the previous structure to follow the guidelines for the training your brain to be ok with leaving food and not finishing everything you consume.

Week 7-8+

The rest of the programme is the same as 'The Master Plan – 26 Week Transformation', as outlined previously.

The Targeted Techniques Plan –

This approach is an unstructured way to address your transformation. With this method you simply apply different techniques to your current routine as dictated by your needs vs your desires.

This can be done in addition to any programme you are doing or simply done without any accompanying plan just to see how it affects your behaviours.

Needs Analysis – What To Focus On?

There are two ways to this approach. One way is to just follow any element that has taken your interest. It could be a previous section resonated with you or you felt you would benefit from a certain technique. In this case pick an exercise from that area and give it a go.

Alternatively, you could look to identify your needs and then focus on the areas of highest priority. To help you with this you can look at the transformation cycle to think about what may help you the most.

Targeted Technique Examples

The unstructured approached could be used as follows;

If you are an emotional eater you may find the best approach for you is to spend the next month focusing on stress reduction. You decide to learn each of the four reduction techniques outlined earlier. You spend one week on each one, doing it for 10 minutes a day to see how it affects your eating.

If motivation is your issue, perhaps you start by using the goal visualisation techniques and learn about creating a relaxed motivation state before eating.

For someone who eats all the time you may decide all you need to do is follow the four behaviour experiments around not eating. Therefore, you practice not finishing the food on your plate and follow this up with the three fasting experiments. This teaches you to be comfortable with changing your eating patterns and not having to eat at any specific time of the day (morning, afternoon or evening). You could do this over the next five weeks while doing your old previous routine.

It could be that you feel your environment is lacking because your friends keep knocking you off track. So you hire a coach, join a cross fit gym and spend three weeks purposefully meeting your friends to learn to be good around food and drink in social situations.

If the history of your body has shown lots of ups and down with your weight you may decide to practice the ability to switch between a fat loss and a maintenance period. Therefore you decide to rotate 3 days fat loss followed by 3 days breakeven for two months.

Creating Your Own Plan of Action

To work out your next step just use the table below as a guide to the techniques you can use. The outline for these details can be found within the previous structured plans.

Motivation	Stress	Plans
Goal Visualisation	Stress Coping	Food Reactions
Goal Priority	Stress Reduction x 4	Food / Step Goals
Goal Environment	Stress Causes	On / Off Weeks
Goal Mood State		

Fitness Personality	Neural
Self-Talk Switching	Leaving Food Exercise
Personal Growth Tasks	Morning Fast
Identity Rules & Imprinting	Day Time Fast
Rituals	Evening Fast
Fitness Environment Techniques	Eating Sensibly Around Friends

This is just a selection of methods within the different areas that can be used. There are many other techniques available within the transformation cycle not outlined here. You may also create your own elements to the plan if you feel it would be helpful.

The Grand Unified Theory of Weight Loss

<u>Your Personalised Plan</u>

This plan is drawing upon all the aspects from the previous three approaches and tailoring it to your own needs. This can mean you select the most necessary elements for you but also put them into a form of structured approach. This is a good method if you enjoy creating your own plan or have access to someone who could put it together for you.

<u>Needs Analysis – The Basis of Plan Creation</u>

The way to optimally structure your plan is through using your own needs and circumstances to decide what techniques should have the highest priority. You should have a good idea of your main needs after reading this far.

<u>Plan Creation Examples</u>

There are no right or wrong ways to set out your plan. It could be you have a holiday in six weeks so you want to get results ASAP. In this case you may use a nutrition plan based on calories and add in daily goal visualisation and stress coping methods so that you can go as hard as possible. After a few weeks you may introduce some fasting methods to bring variety to your eating routine to make it easier to follow.

6 Week Plan		
	Plan – Calorie diet, 1400 /day, 10 000 steps	
Week 1	Goal Visualisations	Stress Reduction
Week 2	Goal Visualisation	Stress Reduction
Week 3	Food Reactions	Goal Mood State
Week 4	Morning Fast	Goal Visualisations
Week 5	Day Fast	Stress Reduction
Week 6	Goal Mood State	Stress Reduction

Longer term plans may use a similar structure to the approaches you have seen previously. However, you may change your order, factor in time off for holidays and switch between using a rigid plans or more relaxed sensible eating patterns with your food. An example of this could look like;

Personalised Transformation Plan – 15 Weeks			
Start	Measurements	Mechanics of Change	
	1	**2**	**3**
1	Sensible Eating	Steps Survey	Stress Reduction
2	Review 1	Goal steps / Eating	Stress Reduction 2
3	Review 2	Morning Fast	Causes of stress
4		Evening Fast	Causes of stress
5	On / Off Days		
6	On / Off days	Day Fast	
7			
8	Formal Diet Plan	Goal Visualisations	
9			
10	Food Reactions	Goal Mood State	
11			
12			
13	Identity Rules	Identity Imprinting	
14	Goal Environment	Rituals	
15	Long Term Structure		

There are an almost endless variety of combinations that can be used so feel free to use your creativity and intuition to come up with a plan to follow. There are also other techniques not outlined here that can be drawn upon to target certain needs or skills.

Troubleshooting & FAQ's

You have now seen four different approaches and structures that can be used to change your body once and for all. Below are some common questions that people ask.

How do I start?

It is easy to get going, first take some measurements as set out in 'Before you start any plan' section. This could just be trying on a goal item of clothing. Then read weeks 1 & 2 of 'The Master Plan'. It is as simple as that.

Once the first two weeks are done, read weeks 3 & 4, everything you need to know is explained. Repeat this process until you have finished the 26 week plan.

All those little questions you probably have are unnecessary 99% of the time. As long as you are being sensible and not harming your body by under eating massively or ignoring warning signs then most questions either do not need to be answered now (the programme will address them later) or are just not important. If you do not get any results in the first two weeks, who cares! Carry on and make the adjustments and eventually you will see changes and make progress.

I cannot lose fat on steps alone, what shall I do?

You <u>can</u> lose fat just walking and moderating food. You just need to give the body a sufficient stimulus. You can do this by either increasing your steps (7 day average) or reducing food intake. Most people normally need to do both. If necessary, you can troubleshoot food intake by counting calories for a few days eating. Your ability to notice changes on your body can be a factor to consider as well.

If you are having problems reducing your food intake to a level that gets results you are not alone so do not worry. This is common. The rest of the programme is designed to develop your ability to do this.

Remember, if you want fast results you can do exercise. It is not banned. The point of the losing fat on steps is that it represents one of the easiest ways to lose fat and puts a rightful emphasis on your nutrition skills. These are linked to the long term likelihood of maintaining your results.

I don't know which plan to do?

Just follow the 26 or 12 week 'Master Plan'. Even if you only do half of it through errors and inconsistencies it is often enough to make significant changes alone. To do the 12 week plan you will need to be fairly motivated. If on the other hand you have no motivation at all, just pick any technique you have read about in the book that appeals to you and try it.

I need to get results FAST! My holiday is in four weeks, what should I do?

Set a calorie based nutrition goal alongside a steps target and add in 1- 7+ exercise sessions a week (unless exercise makes your eating habits worse). With the fat loss stimulus in place add in visualisation techniques to increase motivation and stress reduction methods to reduce distraction.

Can I eat bread?

Yes you can! Take a look at the fat loss myths in section 2 for more on specific food questions. You can have any food or drink you want and still get results. However, you live in the real world so you cannot eat any food in unlimited amounts and still lose fat.

If you happen to be strongly sensitive to bread, or find eating bread causes you to eat too much food overall then maybe you will need to reduce it greatly or completely cut it out.

I cannot do visualisations, what can I do instead?

Yes you can, just sit there and give it a go. You will do some version of a visualisation. Thinking is a form of it and everyone thinks. Most people quit without even trying for five minutes. It is a skill and a technique that develops over time.

Can I just pay a hypnotherapist to do this stuff for me?

It is appealing to think you can just see someone 1 or 2 times and all your problems will disappear. However, real life is not that convenient. Hypnotherapy could have a big benefit or could make no difference whatsoever depending on your underlying needs. This question usually means you do not want to personally engage with this issue or the process of change. Stop that, get involved... it can be fun!

It is impossible to see if I have lost fat, what else can I do? Could I buy a machine or something?

It can be difficult to see changes, especially as your evaluation is influenced by your mood and recent behaviours. While you can buy a machine, unless you have thousands to spend you will not get one accurate enough to completely trust. The most effective way is specific clothes items from your wardrobe that cover both your upper and lower body.

This is so complicated, can you make it simpler?

Yes, forget the theory, just follow the plans as set out here in this section. There is no science or theory in them. Just do the exercises and see what happens over time.

What do you think of Keto? (Any specific diet)

I always get asked what I think of different diets. This may be Keto, Vegan or Atkins. The first thing to understand is that the energy balance equation gets you results. Any nutrition plan is a tool to aid this manipulation. The biggest factor in fat loss is a calorie deficit over time which is down to your behaviours and not any specific type of diet.

Any plan can be used to help you achieve your goals. A good plan has solid foundations in that it tastes good, adapts to your schedule, works for the body, is sustainable and increases adherence and good behaviours across the board. Assuming the plan appeals in the first place then you will only discover if your plan does the other bits by trying it out. The more extreme a plan the more likely it will <u>not</u> work for you. So if you try it and it is not working then just change your plan after you feel you have given it a fair try.

What do you think of Homeopathy, Hypnosis, CBT, Reiki...?

I also get asked a lot about the many types of alternative therapy or therapeutic methods. I am a big fan in general of alternative approaches but it is important to look at any technique and the proposed mechanism by which it will help you. This must match your needs for results.

In general you need to be careful when looking for a magic bullet solution. As you have seen, getting results has many factors interacting with each other. Does the technique address enough of these to get results on it own? This really depends on your situation. The cost of any method should also be a factor, if it low cost both financially and time wise you may as well try it if it already appeals. If it eats up all of your budget and time you would want to really consider how it fits into a multi-faceted approach for results.

I think most techniques have some merit and can help. The power of the placebo effect alone means you could benefit from most methods even if it doesn't work. In general the more stuff you try the greater the potential for learning more about yourself. This can only benefit your results.

How do you approach working with someone?

For me working with a client is a chess match where me and the client are playing against the clients 'bad' side and subconscious. Setting a plan is a delicate balance their needs for results vs what they are actually prepared to do. I only ever ask that someone gives a fair enough effort. I expect people to make all sorts of horrendous mistakes, failures and the like. This is bound to happen and it is expected. I never get annoyed or lose patience with someone as long as they are trying. Sometimes I start with a formal nutrition plan, other times focusing on stress. It depends on them and if I am working online or face to face. I try to make it as simple as possible yet targeting the areas to give the best results.

Can you just give me some simple stuff to do to get started?

There are all kinds of simple things you could start with almost zero effort. Some of these include; reduce the size of the dishes you eat from, slow down your eating (put the fork or food down between mouthfuls), download an app and meditate before bed, walk before work and after even if for a short period of time, count your calories and steps for a week, think about your goal for 1 minute after you brush your teeth, plan your next meal while eating your current meal, arrange a weekly walk with friends. There are so many things you could do, just pick one and start then see what happens. It is as easy as that.

*****

Many questions I receive are basically individual questions about your own circumstances, here are some answers to common situations that you may find apply to you.

The whole point of the Grand Unified Theory of Body Transformations is that there are different needs for each person so all the answers below are just a guestimate and generalisation of your situation so adapt it as necessary.

I have depression, what should I do?

When suffering any mental health issue, you will need to accept that there are going to be good and bad phases. In a bad phase you will look to just get through it any which way you can. If you can roughly break even then that is great as when you are back in a better functioning phase you can look to make progress. If not, there is no need to beat yourself up.

Ideally during the better periods you will look to put in place things that will help decrease the frequency and severity of the down periods. The actual process outside of this may not be hugely different to anyone else trying to get in shape.

Depression is affected by many things, for some it is a chemical issue within the body (needs medical support). For others it is the physical stimulus given to the body (sleep dis-regulation, sensitive foods, alcohol, lack of exercise). Finally, it can be caused from emotional issues (stress, trauma, current state of your life). Your depression could be affected by one or all of these issues.

Many of these possible factors are addressed within the unified transformation cycle so you may find changing your body has a positive influence on the severity or frequency of depression. As with any medical issue, you should be in consultation with a doctor during the process.

I am severely overweight, what should I do?

Start slow and be patient, your long term success should be about changing who you are as a person primarily and this takes time. Too often people who are very overweight are just lectured about what to eat or how to move. However, what if you simply do not enjoy the feeling of moving or find the warmth of food comforting when you are stressed? That does not make you a bad person or mean anything negative about you. However, it does make it a little harder to get in shape.

The way to start your approach is by thinking about your needs. What do you need to do to enjoy moving? How can you enjoy the taste of food but reduce the overall intake amount? How else can you find comfort without eating? There have been many options shown for doing all of these things in the book. So I would say do one cycle of the master plan set out previously and see where it takes you. Throughout it all, be patient and kind to yourself.

I drink wine every night, what should I do?

This comes back to a personal choice in regards to what to do with the wine. In transformation terms you can usually achieve your goals while still drinking, just look at it in calorie terms and get the energy balance equation to match. To do this though, be wary of any foods consumed alongside the alcohol itself as this can greatly increase energy intake.

My usual advice is to ensure you are choosing to drink, that means you can just as easily say no to a drink as saying yes in any situation. This may be when you are alone on a Tuesday or out on Saturday with friends. To get to this state you will need to do some behaviour experiments while you are motivated to purposely abstain at a time / place you would usually drink.

There are good books on the subject of not drinking such as Rational Recovery by Jack Trimpey (1996), The Sober Diaries by Clare Pooley (2018) and many more. There are also Addiction programmes such as Alcoholic Anonymous.

If you are drinking large amounts of alcohol per day then there is a safety concern to discuss with your doctor about stopping and going cold turkey.

My back and ankle hurt when I move, what can I do?

Injuries can be a real block to creating momentum. The good news is that an exercise rehabilitation programme if structured well can get rid of most typical pains.

A rehab plan works through stretching specific tight areas, employing massage in overly tense parts and strengthening weak muscles. There are numerous elements to this process but most aches and pains can be resolved. There are various online sources available on the net. If you are very sedentary then many pains clear up from simple exercise.

While in the process of rehabilitating injuries you would need to modify your movement routine to allow for your injuries. This could be making use of a stationary bike if unable to walk or if completely unable to move then greatly reducing your food intake. To still receive the mental benefits of exercise it is advised to do any exercise form still available to you that does not affect the injury, e.g. stretching, upper body work.

You would then go through the process as set out previously. As you can always lose body fat if you reduce your food intake, if movement is greatly reduced you can focus more on the things that influence eating, e.g. goal visualisations, reducing stress, adding taste to lower calorie foods etc.

I am Pregnant, What Can I Do?

When you are pregnant it is <u>not</u> the time to be looking to lose body fat. However, it is still a great opportunity to make some progress around your healthy behaviours. You can sensibly work on some of your connections around junk food, focus on gentle movement patterns or develop your awareness around healthy eating. However, the plans in this book are <u>not</u> set out for pregnancy so I would not follow them.

I want to win a bikini show, do you think it is possible?

If you want to win a physique show (bikini, body fitness, fitness model, classic bodybuilding etc.) then make sure you know what is required of you.

It is certainly possible to compete and win, someone has to, but it certainly is not easy nor a fast process. Personally, I think your attitude is wrong to start with. The desire to win a show before you entered the sport is a little ahead of time.

In my experience, out of all the people who I have heard talk about winning a show before they have actually competed only a tiny fraction ever actually got on stage. The fear of losing is part of this reason. Your first time on stage should be about the achievement of doing something so few people ever would do, if you come home with a trophy then well done but anyone up there is a winner. If you are serious about winning you will need a coach. There is almost no chance you will win one on your own without specialised knowledge.

As for the requirements, it takes up your whole life. You will need a stable life in general as the lifestyle is very regimented. You will need to train daily for years. Your food structure will be similar day in day out. Almost no one drinks who competes and their social life is heavily based around the gym.

Though to be fair, this it is not a million miles away from how a very active person acts. So a little of this depends on your current background.

You need to consider your history around food and your body. Nothing can agitate a food disorder or body image issue quicker than physique competitions. If you have a history of bad eating patterns it may not be for you. I would personally get into crazy good shape first before truly considering if you want to compete on stage. You should also go and watch a couple of shows live and chat to people who have already been involved with the sport.

I have a history of eating disorders, what should I do?

We have touched on some eating disorder issues at a very surface level already though it is a little beyond the scope of the book. There is a point with eating disorders where you should work with a professional in the field so ensure you have considered this. With that said I have worked with and seen people make great strides in this area.

I would tackle any food issue separately to trying to change your body. For example, if you want to reduce your binge eating, focus on it when you are <u>not</u> trying to lose fat. If you insist on losing fat you need to do it very slowly and also take regular breaks to return to break even.

It is also important to have clear criteria around when your eating behaviours are not at an appropriate level and are becoming more disordered. This allows you to check in to see if your plan to change your body is causing unwanted side effects around your eating patterns etc.

We are on lockdown due to Coronavirus, What can I do?

There are a few things you can to try to offset the impact of the lockdown. Depending on your restrictions you should implement some of the following.

If you are allowed out to exercise or walk then I would immediately begin commuting to work even though you are probably working at home. Replicate your old commute time by walking for 30 to 60 minutes around your local area before and after your work day. Other options include looking to combine walking with any work calls that do not need you to be at the computer. If you are unable to leave the house, or prefer to stay indoors then renting or buying exercise equipment can be a great idea. You can gently exercise on a treadmill, rower or stationary bike while watching TV or listening to work conference calls. For general movement you do not need to walk fast or exercise hard to get the benefits.

Alongside your movement you would want to impose some structure around your food and eating. As you are at home you can eat anytime you want and this lack of a regime can lead to you eating a lot more food. To counter this, set some meal times for you to eat. If you are now moving much less than before due to the restrictions then you will need to reduce your food intake as well. The simplest way to do this would be to eat fewer meals per day and/or cutting out snacking between meals.

Being at home all the time can greatly increase stress levels, especially as some of your stress releases have probably been taken away. You should expand upon your use of the stress management methods outlined previously. This could mean daily meditations, learning Emotional Freedom Technique or online counselling. You may also want to increase your own self-care practice during these times.

It is important to culture an environment that supports being active and healthy. There are many subtle things that can prevent this, for example, whether you get dressed properly every morning or instead stay in the clothes that you slept in. You would want to implement as many measures as possible that improve your behaviours. This could include getting up at the same time every day, immediately getting dressed into your sports gear or reducing the size of your plates to encourage smaller quantities. It could mean you join an online fitness class of some sort so you are at least around other active people even if just virtually. Maybe you could start meeting a friend to exercise if allowed within the rules. It can also help greatly if you work with a coach in some form.

You should also test and challenge your beliefs. Lockdowns in the winter are much tougher than the summer due to the conditions. Maybe you will need to learn to go outside in the rain or exercise earlier in the morning to maximise daylight. With the right clothes you will find it is not as bad as you think weather wise and that your body soon adapts to earlier exercise or any other changes you may implement.

While lockdown is tough it also is a great opportunity to get results. A large amount of people have managed to get amazing results during it. You may find you actually have more time than before to dedicate to movement. It is also possible you have less negative influences around food and drink due to your reduced social life.

If you do gain weight during this period then do not beat yourself up. It is not the end of the world. Your primary concern should be just to get through this. You can always change your body in the future so relax. This kind of upheaval will probably never happen again in your lifetime so just do the best that you can and be kind to yourself.

Final Message

I hope you are inspired to take action and know that you can achieve your goals. There is nothing that can stop you being successful if you commit to a holistic and varied approach as outlined in this book. To unlock your potential you should start today and then persist onwards. Make use of what you have learnt and you will soon see the results.

I look forward to hearing about what you achieve.

To your success!

Ben Wilson

Further Reading –

The following books are recommended for further reading as they expand on many of the elements within the Grand Unified Theory. There are so many different contributing areas this is not an exhaustive list.

-**Atomic Habits: An Easy & Proven Way to Build Good Habits & Break Bad Ones** Paperback – 18 Oct. 2018 by James Clear (Author) Random House Business

-**Intuitive Eating**, 4th Edition: A Revolutionary Anti-Diet Approach Paperback – Illustrated, 23 Jun. 2020 by Evelyn Tribole (Author), Essentials; Illustrated Edition

-**Never Enough: The Neuroscience and Experience of Addiction** (The Addicted Brain) Paperback – 8 Aug. 2019 by Judith Grisel (Author), Scribe UK

-**Never Binge Again: Reprogram Yourself to Think Like a Permanently Thin Person. Stop Overeating and Binge Eating and Stick to the Food Plan of Your Choice**! Paperback – 25 Aug. 2015 by Glenn Livingston Ph.D. (Author) CreateSpace Independent Publishing Platform

-**Out Of The Shadows: Understanding Sexual Addiction** Paperback – Illustrated, 12 Jan. 2018 by Patrick J. Carnes (Author) Hazelden Trade

-**Psycho-Cybernetics**, Updated and Expanded Paperback – 3 Nov. 2015 by Maxwell Maltz (Author) Perigee Books

-**Rational Recovery: The New Cure for Substance Addiction** Paperback – Illustrated, 1 Nov. 1996 by Jack Trimpey (Author) Pocket Books

-**The Brain over Binge Recovery Guide: A Simple and Personalized Plan for Ending Bulimia and Binge Eating Disorder** Paperback – 11 Jan. 2016 by Kathryn Hansen (Author), Camellia Publishing

-**The Body Keeps the Score: Mind, Brain and Body in the Transformation of Trauma** Paperback – 24 Sept. 2015 by Bessel van der Kolk (Author) Penguin

-**The Talent Code: Greatness isn't born. It's grown** Paperback – 4 Mar. 2010 by Daniel Coyle (Author) Arrow

-**The Hungry Brain: Outsmarting the Instincts That Make Us Overeat** Paperback – 6 April 2017 by Dr Stephan Guyenet (Author) Vermilion

-**Thinking, Fast and Slow** Paperback – 10 May 2012 by Daniel Kahneman (Author), Penguin

-**Why We Sleep: The New Science of Sleep and Dreams** Paperback – 4 Jan. 2018 by Matthew Walker (Author) Penguin

-**Words That Change Minds: The 14 Patterns for Mastering the Language of Influence Paperback** – 2019 by Shelle Rose Charvet (Author), Bloomanity

References

1) Dr. Abravanel's Body Type Diet and Lifetime Nutrition Plan - Elliot D. Abravanel, Elizabeth A. King. 1999

2) Female Figure Identifcation Techniques (FFIT) For Apparel – Simmons, Istook, Devarajan, 2004

   Summary of the eight types -
   https://shopyourshape.com/body-shapes/

3) Science ABC – Scientific Analysis of Michael Philips's Body Type - 2019

   https://www.scienceabc.com/sports/michael-phelps-height-arms-torso-arm-span-feet-swimming.html

4) These graphs are my representation of the data from using data from government sources, such as:

   Statistics on Obesity, Physical Activity and Diet, England, 2020 –
   https://digital.nhs.uk/data-and-information/publications/statistical/statistics-on-obesity-physical-activity-and-diet/england-2020

   Health Survey For England -
   https://digital.nhs.uk/data-and-information/publications/statistical/health-survey-for-england/2017

5) Body fat data is my interpretation as compiled from BMI estimated using the relationship between body fat and BMI as seen in many research and obesity discussions such as:

Association between physical activity and body fat percentage, with adjustment for BMI: a large cross-sectional analysis of UK Biobank
Bradbury, Guo, Cairns, Armstrong, Key, 2016
https://bmjopen.bmj.com/content/7/3/e011843

Body Fat Percentage Comparison Calculator for Men and Women in the United States
https://dqydj.com/body-fat-percentage-distribution-men-women/

The association between physical activity and body fat percentage with adjustment for body mass index in China:
Zou, Su,Du, Ouyang, Wang, Wang, Ding, Zhang, 2015

https://bmcpublichealth.biomedcentral.com/articles/10.1186/s12889-020-08832-0

6) Hannah Ritchie (2017) - "Obesity".
https://ourworldindata.org/obesity

Obesity Update 2017 – OCED :
http://www.oecd.org/health/health-systems/Obesity-Update-2017.pdf

7) Four Decades of Obesity Trends among Non-Hispanic Whites and Blacks in the United States:
C. Mary Schooling, 2016
https://www.ncbi.nlm.nih.gov/pmc/articles/PMC5125692/

Perspectives from United Kingdom and United States Policy Makers on Obesity Prevention: Workshop Summary.
Institute of Medicine (US) Standing Committee on Childhood Obesity Prevention, 2010
https://www.ncbi.nlm.nih.gov/books/NBK220230/

8) Ethnicity-Related Skeletal Muscle Differences Across the Lifespan
Silva, Shen, Heo, Gallagher, Wang, Sardinha, Heymsfield - 2010
https://www.ncbi.nlm.nih.gov/pmc/articles/PMC2795070/

9) Physical activity in adults
Health Survey For England 2016
http://healthsurvey.hscic.gov.uk/media/63730/HSE16-Adult-phy-act.pdf

Fitness industry in the United Kingdom (UK) - Statistics & Facts – Statista
David Lange, 2019

https://www.statista.com/topics/3411/fitness-industry-in-the-united-kingdom-uk/

10) Experiencing Physical Warmth Promotes
Interpersonal Warmth
Lawrence E. Williams and John A. Bargh
https://science.sciencemag.org/content/sci/suppl/2008/10/23/322.5901.606.DC1/Williams.SOM.pdf

11) Resistance to exercise-induced weight loss:
compensatory behavioral adaptations
Melanson, Keadle, Donnelly, Braun, King - 2014
https://www.ncbi.nlm.nih.gov/pmc/articles/PMC3696411/

12) Toxicological Function of Adipose Tissue: Focus on
Persistent Organic Pollutants

La Merrill, Emond, Kim, Antignac, Le Bizec, Clément,
Birnbaum, Barouki, 2013

https://www.ncbi.nlm.nih.gov/pmc/articles/PMC3569688/

13) Structure of Adipose Tissue -
https://en.wikipedia.org/wiki/Adipose_tissue

Structure of Body Fat (Triglyceride) -
https://en.wikipedia.org/wiki/Lipolysis

14) Calorie Definition -
https://en.wikipedia.org/wiki/Calorie

15) Effect of exercise intensity, duration and mode on post-exercise oxygen consumption
https://pubmed.ncbi.nlm.nih.gov/14599232/

16) Calorie & Macro data from Nutrition Data -
https://nutritiondata.self.com/

17) Energy Metabolism, Fuel Selection and Body Weight Regulation
J Galgani and E Ravussin, 2008
https://www.ncbi.nlm.nih.gov/pmc/articles/PMC2897177/

18) Metabolic and Behavioral Compensatory Responses to Exercise Interventions: Barriers to Weight Loss
King, Caudwell, Hopkins, Byrne, Colley, Hills, Stubbs, Blundell (2012)
https://onlinelibrary.wiley.com/doi/full/10.1038/oby.2007.164

19) The role of leptin and ghrelin in the regulation of food intake and body weight in humans: a review
Klok Jakobsdottir Drent (2006)
https://onlinelibrary.wiley.com/doi/full/10.1111/j.1467-789X.2006.00270.x

20) S ports & Exercise Nutrition – Mc Ardle, Katch & Katch
1999, Lippincott Williams & Wilkins

Glycogen storage capacity and de novo lipogenesis
during massive carbohydrate overfeeding in man
Acheson , Schutz, Bessard, Anantharaman, Flatt,
Jéquier, 1988
https://pubmed.ncbi.nlm.nih.gov/3165600/

Fasting substrate oxidation at rest assessed by
indirect calorimetry: is prior dietary macronutrient
level and composition a confounder?

Miles-Chan, Dulloo & Schutz
International Journal of Obesity volume 39, (2015)
https://www.nature.com/articles/ijo201529#Tab1

21) The Effects of Overfeeding on Body Composition: The
Role of Macronutrient Composition – A Narrative
Review

LEAF, ANTONIO, 2017

https://www.ncbi.nlm.nih.gov/pmc/articles/PMC578
6199/

Fat and carbohydrate overfeeding in humans:
different effects on energy storage

Horton, Drougas, Brachey, Reed, Peters, Hill

The American Journal of Clinical Nutrition, 1995,
Pages 19–29,

https://pubmed.ncbi.nlm.nih.gov/7598063/

22) Role of Energy Excretion in Human Body Weight Regulation
Lund, Gerhart-Hines, Clemmensen, 2020
https://doi.org/10.1016/j.tem.2020.06.002

23) Walking Energy Calculator
https://www.omnicalculator.com/sports/walking-calorie

24) Is an Energy Surplus Required to Maximize Skeletal Muscle Hypertrophy Associated With Resistance Training
Slater, Dieter, Marsh, Helms, Shaw, Iraki, 2019
https://www.ncbi.nlm.nih.gov/pmc/articles/PMC6710320/

25) National Institute For Health and Clinical Excellence - Weight management before, during and after pregnancy
https://www.nice.org.uk/guidance/PH27

26) International Society of Sports Nutrition Position Stand: protein and exercise
https://pubmed.ncbi.nlm.nih.gov/28642676/

27) The Effects of Supraphysiological Doses of Testosterone on muscle size and strength in normal men N England. J. Med., 335:1, 1996,

Anabolic steroids: the physiological effects of placebos ARIEL, GIDEON; SAVILLE, WILLIAM Medicine and Science in Sports: July 1972 - Volume 4 - Issue 2 - p 124-126

28) Food Allergies – The Basics Valenta, Hochwallner, Linhart, Pahr, 2015 https://www.ncbi.nlm.nih.gov/pmc/articles/PMC4414527/

https://www.medicinenet.com/what_are_the_four_types_of_allergic_reactions/article.htm

29) Consequences of physical inactivity in older adults: A systematic review of reviews and meta-analyses

Cunningham , O' Sullivan, Caserotti , Tully

https://pubmed.ncbi.nlm.nih.gov/32020713/

30) Biochemical Individuality: Basis for the Genetotrophic Concept - Roger Williams

31) Sales Brain Neuro-Marketing
https://www.salesbrain.com/

32) Personality Types & Systems -
https://en.wikipedia.org/wiki/Personality_type

33) 5 Cycling Weight Loss Successes -
https://www.bicycling.com/health-
nutrition/a20025027/5-cycling-weight-loss-successes/

34) Features of a successful therapeutic fast of 382 days'
duration - 125kg lost in one year

Stewart and Fleming, 1973,
https://www.ncbi.nlm.nih.gov/pmc/articles/PMC249
5396/?page=1

David Goggins 48kg in 12 weeks - Can't Hurt Me:
Master Your Mind and Defy the Odds - David Goggins,
Lioncrest Publishing, 2018

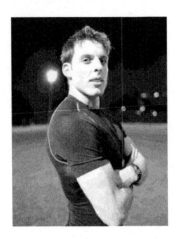

Ben Wilson –

Ben is a Personal Trainer, Nutritionist and Behavioural Change Coach who has been helping people lose weight and get into shape since 2002.

He has studied various behaviour change and stress management strategies. These include Emotional Freedom Technique (EFT) and Neuro-linguistic programming (NLP). He wrote the book "Change Your Thinking, Change Your Shape" (2011) which looked at the thoughts and beliefs that promote success when transforming your body.

In addition to this he possesses a degree in Chemistry from the University of Cardiff and studied personalised nutrition through Metabolic Typing and Functional Diagnostic Nutrition. A qualified personal trainer his studies in strength and conditioning led him to write the book 'Rugby Fitness Training: A Twelve Month Conditioning Programme' (2006).

A regular in the media Ben has made numerous TV and Radio appearances. He has been on BBC 1. Sky TV, CNN News and many other media outlets.

Connect With Me

You can reach me on most social media at – Benwilsonuk

www.Instagram.com/benwilsonuk

www.facebook.com/benwilsonuk

www.youtube.com/benwilsonuk1

I send out recaps of my latest videos, articles and free gifts through my website newsletter. This builds on more of the themes discussed in this book. Join it at:

www.benwilsonuk.com/news/

For more information on my programmes and coaching check out my website for more details.

Printed in Great Britain
by Amazon

41389801R00245